The Year Before Death

CLIVE SEALE
Department of Sociology
Goldsmiths College
University of London

ANN CARTWRIGHT
Institute for Social Studies in Medical Care
London

Avebury
Aldershot · Brookfield USA · Hong Kong · Singapore · Sydney

© C. Seale and A. Cartwright, 1994

All rights reserved. No part of this publication may be reproduced, stored in a retrieval system, or transmitted in any form or by any means, electronic, mechanical, photocopying or otherwise without the prior permission of the publisher.

Published by
Avebury
Ashgate Publishing Limited
Gower House
Croft Road
Aldershot
Hants GU11 3HR
England

Ashgate Publishing Company
Old Post Road
Brookfield
Vermont 05036
USA

British Library Cataloguing in Publication Data

Seale, Clive
　　The Year Before Death
　　I. Title II. Cartwright, Ann
　　306.9

ISBN 1 85628 604 5

Printed and Bound in Great Britain by
Athenaeum Press Ltd, Newcastle upon Tyne.

Contents

Tables	vii
Acknowledgements	xiv
1 Introduction	1
2 Changes since 1969	18
Part I: The experience of illness, death and bereavement	29
Introduction	31
3 Communication and awareness	34
4 Religious belief	52
5 The experience of caring	62
6 Social class differences	77
7 Old age	87
Part II: Hospice, hospital and institutional care	95
Introduction	97
8 The experience of hospice care	100

9	Hospices in context	112
10	Hospitals	124
11	Residential and nursing homes	130
12	Day centres (written by Graham Farrow)	147

Part III: Care in the community — 161

Introduction — 163

13	The balance of care	166
14	General practitioners	175
15	Community nurses	195
16	The relationship between professionals	210
17	Conclusion	219

Bibliography — 225

Copyright acknowledgements — 235

Index — 237

Tables

Table 1.1	Hospice services in England and Wales (1969-93)	1
Table 1.2	Percentage of elderly people in the population by gender (England and Wales)	3
Table 1.3	Elderly persons per general practitioner (UK) 1951-90	4
Table 1.4	Percentage of NHS general practitioner consultations by site (Great Britain)	5
Table 1.5	Changes in the district nursing service: 1972-87/8 (England)	5
Table 1.6	Meals, home helps and chiropody: 1969-87 (England)	6
Table 1.7	People aged 65+ in residential homes 1969-87	7
Table 1.8	Study areas for "The year before death in 1987"	12
Table 1.9	Sample sizes and response rates: 1987 study	14
Table 1.10	Respondent's relationship to the person who died	15

Table 2.1	Age at death and place of death in 1969 and 1987 samples	19
Table 2.2	Household composition	19
Table 2.3	Length of time in hospital or other institutions in the year before death	20
Table 2.4	General practitioner consultations in year before death	21
Table 2.5	Symptoms reported in 1969 and 1987 for cancer and other deaths	23
Table 2.6	Dying person's knowledge of condition and prognosis	25
Table 2.7	Proportion of respondents who felt the dying peoples' knowledge or lack of knowledge about the prognosis was "best as it was"	26
Table 3.1	Respondents' knowledge of condition and prognosis	39
Table 3.2	Original respondents' and deceaseds' knowledge about whether the person would die	41
Table 3.3	People who knew what was wrong with them and that they would die: professionals who told them, by condition and year	43
Table 3.4	Respondents who knew what was wrong and that the person would die: professionals who told them by condition and year	44
Table 3.5	People who knew what was wrong and that death would result: who told the deceased and the original respondent (1987)	45
Table 3.6	Who respondent talked to about the deceased's illness and what might happen	50

Table 4.1	Variations with nature of faith or denomination	53
Table 4.2	Age at death and belief in some sort of life after death	54
Table 4.3	Variations with religious faith in acceptance and discussion of death	56
Table 4.4	Association between relatives' and deceaseds' religious faiths	58
Table 4.5	Beliefs of relatives and deceased about some sort of life after death	58
Table 4.6	Variation in reported quality of relationship between relative and the person who died with the religious faith of the relative	60
Table 5.1	Household composition by family composition, restrictions, age, sex, marital status, cause of death and where lived (1987)	64
Table 5.2	Restrictions reported for people who spent some part of their last year at home (sudden deaths under 65 excluded)	66
Table 5.3	Who bore the brunt of caring for those with restrictions, by household composition	68
Table 5.4	Adjustment to death	73
Table 6.1	Social class differences in health, care and circumstances in the year before death	78
Table 7.1	Variations with age at death	88
Table 7.2	Symptoms for which no difference with age at death reported and proportion for whom symptom reported	90
Table 7.3	Symptoms with an age variation	90

Table 7.4	Problems with housing by age at death	91
Table 7.5	Proportion receiving care from home help services by age at death and whether living alone (excluding those in residential homes for year before death)	92
Table 8.1	Respondents' views about the degree of reassurance and support provided by domiciliary nurses	104
Table 8.2	Respondents' views of the care from doctors during in-patient stays	107
Table 8.3	Respondents' views about nursing care during in-patient stays	107
Table 9.1	Proportion of deaths from cancer, by age	114
Table 9.2	Sex, family and place of residence by cause of death and age	114
Table 9.3	Symptoms reported as experienced in the last 12 months of life in a sample of 639 adults by cause of death and age	115
Table 9.4	Restrictions experienced at home by a sample of adults in the last 12 months of life, by age and cause	116
Table 9.5	Experience of long term restriction, by age and cause	117
Table 9.6	Knowledge of diagnosis and awareness of likely death, by age and cause	120
Table 9.7	Views about the time of death, by cause and age (excluding sudden deaths)	121
Table 10.1	Age at death and use of hospital or hospice service	125

Table 10.2	Cause of death and use of hospital or hospice service	126
Table 11.1	Length of time spent in different types of home	131
Table 11.2	Characteristics of people spending some or all of last year of their lives in residential homes	132
Table 11.3	Symptoms reported more often for people in residential homes	135
Table 11.4	Consultations, home visits and night calls in the last 12 months of their lives for those living in residential homes and others under the care of general practitioners	136
Table 11.5	Variations in proportion admitted to hospital in the last year of their lives with stay in residential homes	138
Table 11.6	Views of relatives, friends or neighbours on various aspects of the home	140
Table 11.7	Quality of life analyzed by time in residential home for those for whom relative responded	144
Table 12.1	Age, sex, marital status and household composition by day centre attendance in the last year of life	149
Table 12.2	Experience of long term restriction by day centre attendance in the last year of life	150
Table 12.3	Experience of long term symptoms by attendance at a day centre in the last year of life	151
Table 12.4	What did he/she do at the day centre?	153

Table 13.1	Views on balance of care for the dying	167
Table 13.2	Views on further facilities needed in their area	167
Table 13.3	Availability of community services and views on whether they should be introduced or extended	169
Table 13.4	Doctors' views about proportion of instances in which pain in dying patients can be satisfactorily controlled	172
Table 14.1	Contacts with general practitioners in the last year of life	176
Table 14.2	Variation in the number of home visits and night calls with age during the last year of life	177
Table 14.3	Proportion of general practitioners wanting more training in various aspects of terminal care by whether or not they would like to be able to give more time to patients who are dying	186
Table 14.4	Relationship between doctors' own emotional reactions to death and dying and views on further training	188
Table 14.5	Estimated number of home visits and other consultations for patients of doctors with different list sizes	189
Table 14.6	Variation with doctor's age in respondents' assessments of the doctor and his or her care	190
Table 15.1	Type of nurse involved at each stage: original respondents, general views and specific patient questionnaires	196

Table 15.2	Visiting patterns of district nurses reported by original respondents: 1969 and 1987	198
Table 15.3	Adequacy of communication with hospitals and general practitioners judged by community nurses: 1969 and 1987	201
Table 16.1	Availability of specialist domiciliary services and views on whether they should be introduced or extended	214
Table 16.2	Views on helpfulness of specialist domiciliary advice on symptom relief for terminal care by whether service available in their area	216

Acknowledgements

We are particularly grateful to the relatives and friends of the people who died who answered our many questions, often recalling sad and poignant memories to do so. We are also greatly indebted to the general practitioners, consultants and nurses who participated in the study and to the administrators, managers and staff who helped us to identify the doctors and nurses.

Many others contributed to the study: The Office of Population Censuses and Surveys, particularly Pat Hunter and Maureen Hoskins, who provided the sample of deaths; the interviewers on the main and pilot study - Helen Allen, Tessa Bain, Jenny Bell, Irene Boller, Gillian Calder, Sheila Chetham, Joan Gallop, Hilary Gellman, Hilary Golden, Margaret Jones, Josephine Leighton, Jane Malone, Kay Morley, Caroline Morris, Marie Oxtoby, Joan Read, Rita Redston, Ellen Southwell, Jenny Spackman, Ann Start, Ron Thompson, Amanda Thurstone, Gillian Wall, Barbara Walton and Joan Worthington; the coders - Dorothy Goodwin and Margaret Hall; for data entry - Hazel Adams; for statistical and computing help Joy Windsor; for secretarial help - Heather Taylor and Brenda Griffiths; for financial control - Louis Hancock; for research assistance - Graham Farrow; other colleagues who contributed in a variety of ways - Nick Baker, David Field, Juliet Formby, Irene Higginson, Ann Jacoby, Emma Jefferys, Kathryn McCann, Mark McCarthy, Caroline Plimley, Isabelle Seale, Ian Sinclair, Sue Tester, Alwyn Turner and Pat Webb; David Metcalf and David Wilkin at the Centre for Primary Care Research in Manchester who gave us hospitality for our briefings; Colin Murray Parkes who tried to persuade two ethical committees to approve the study; the members of the Institute's Advisory Committee - Abe Adelstein, Tony Alment, Val Beral, Vera Carstairs, May Clarke, Karen Dunnell, John Fox, Austin Heady, Margot Jefferys, Joyce Leeson, John McEwan, Martin Richards, Alwyn Smith, Mike Wadsworth and Jenny

Griffin; the Department of Health who gave us additional information about general practitioners and funded AC's salary and the Institute overheads. The Medical Research Council funded CS's salary and the costs of the study.

The publishers of various journals, in which many of the chapters of this book first appeared as articles, generously gave their permission for us to reprint the material. A full listing of the articles and their sources is given at the very end of the book.

We are grateful to them all.

1 Introduction

Over the past 25 years death, and the care of people who are dying, have increasingly become matters of public discussion, so that it is often said that death is no longer a taboo topic. Alongside this change, and contributing to it, has been the growth of the modern hospice movement (see Table 1.1), which began with the founding of St Christopher's Hospice in London in 1967. This movement, which has a self-avowedly educational mission, spread widely, through North America, Australia and other countries during the 1970s and 1980s.

Less spectacularly, there have been changes in the United Kingdom in the provision and structure of other services available to those who are dying, including the hospital service, primary medical care and domiciliary nursing and social services. Underlying this has been a mood amongst policy makers

Table 1.1
Hospice services in England and Wales (1969-93)

	In-patient units	Beds	Home care teams	Hospital support	Day care
1969	17*	-	1	0	0
1987	106	1983	167	23	58
1993	166	2516	348	179	177

* Most of these were nursing homes caring for the terminally ill.

Source: Lunt and Hillier 1981; St Christopher's Hospice Information Service 1987, 1993.

(shared in the experience of many other nations) which intensified with the oil crisis of the early 1970s, of concern about public expenditure on welfare services, in which the provision of resources for care of elderly people has been seen as an increasingly heavy burden (Victor 1991).

At the same time there have been changes in the demographic profile of those who are near to death, which influences the type of care that they need and receive. In many Western and other industrialised societies there has been an increase in the proportion of elderly people, and in particular of elderly people with diminished resources for care.

This book is about the impact of these changes on the situation of people who die, particularly in the period between 1969 and 1987, the dates of the two research studies that are the focus of the book. The purpose of both studies was to describe the last year of life of a randomly selected sample of adults who had died. It is not a book primarily about terminal care, but about the circumstances of people who die. One of our chief arguments in this book is that there has been, over the past 20 years or so, a tendency for those who specialise in terminal care to dominate public discussion of the care of the dying. However, not everyone who dies is considered by themselves or those around them, to be dying - except in the sense that we are all moving towards our deaths. It will become clear that this distinction - between terminal illness and life before death - is important in giving a truly representative account of the circumstances of people who die.

In addition to issues that are of concern to those providing services to people who die, an important purpose of this book is to describe the variety of ways in which the last year of life may be experienced. This is because old age and death is a matter of general human concern, as we all die. Some of us may be somewhat unwilling to contemplate it, others curious to know what the experience of dying might be like. This book shows the great diversity of circumstances of people in their last year, and describes both their situation and the experiences and feelings of friends, family and others who knew them, and in many cases looked after them, in their final illness.

This introductory chapter provides a brief overview of the more important changes over the past two decades or so that impinge on peoples' experience of the last year of life. In addition, the methods of the studies on which this book is based will be described, and an indication given of its structure.

Demographic change

There has, throughout the twentieth century, been a gradual increase in longevity and in the proportion of the population that can be considered "elderly". This has particularly adverse implications for the care of elderly women once they become dependant. Life expectancy in the UK, as well as most other industrialised countries, is longer for women. In 1969 in England and Wales, life expectancy at birth for men was 68.5, for women 74.8; by 1987 this had risen to 72.6 for men and 78.3 for women (Office of Health Economics 1992). In addition, women tend to marry men who are older. A large proportion of the elderly, and particularly of the very old (85+) are therefore elderly widows (Arber and Ginn 1991). Table 1.2 shows changes between 1969 and 1987 in the elderly proportion of the population.

The household structure of the elderly has been increasingly characterised by a decline in the numbers of those living with others, and an increase in living alone. Dale et al. (1987) report that whereas 10 per cent of the elderly (65+) population lived alone in 1945, this figure was 34 per cent by 1980. Of those living in private households, 48 per cent of women aged 65+ and 20 per cent of men of this age lived alone in 1987 (OPCS 1989a). In addition, almost twice as many women as men enter institutional care. Thus in the 1981 Census 4.6 per cent of women aged 65+ lived in "communal establishments" (which include long stay hospitals, nursing and residential homes) but only 2.5 per cent of men in this age bracket (Arber and Ginn 1991).

The ability of elderly people to cope with the dependency that is brought by illness and disability is affected by their access to both material resources and resources supplied by carers. Arber and Ginn (1991) show that elderly women are significantly disadvantaged on both these fronts. Thus in 1989 almost twice as many women as men aged 65+ claimed Income Support, an indicator of poverty (Arber and Ginn 1991), an important reason for this inequality in income being the lack of an occupational pension for many women. In addition, due to their family and living circumstances, elderly women dependent on care are less likely to be looked after by spouses and are more dependent on state provided domiciliary services.

Table 1.2
Percentage of elderly people in the population by gender (England and Wales)

	Proportion of population aged:			
	65+		75+	
Year	Men	Women	Men	Women
1969	10.2%	15.6%	3.1%	6.1%
1987	12.8%	18.4%	4.7%	8.7%

Source: OPCS (1977, 1993)

These demographic changes have profound consequences for many people in their last year of life. Dying, for many people, is the final phase of a longer experience of old age. The circumstances of those who die in large part reflect the general position of the elderly in society.

Changes in general practice

Since 1969 there have been a number of significant changes in the provision of general practitioner services which are likely to have impinged on the care of those in their last year of life. There has been a growth in the proportion of general practitioners who practice in a health centre, or in group practices rather than single handed. The proportion of single handed practitioners declined from 22% in 1969 (DHSS 1973) to 11.5% in 1987 (DoH 1989), meaning that it was more likely at the later date that sick people would receive care from more than one family doctor. In addition, list sizes have declined as the proportion of doctors to the population has risen. Thus in 1969 the average list size in England was 2,495; by 1987 it was 2,010 (DHSS 1982 and Office of Health Economics 1992). This might suggest that those in the last year of life could expect more services from general practitioners, but an examination of coverage according to the age group of those served suggests otherwise. Table 1.3 shows that the numbers very elderly (75+ and 85+) per general practitioner has steadily increased since 1951. This is due to the increase in numbers of the elderly outstripping the increase in numbers of general practitioners. Since older people also consult their general practitioners more frequently (OPCS 1989a) it is unlikely that

Table 1.3
Elderly persons per general practitioner* (UK) 1951-90

Year	65+	75+	85+
1951	271	88	11
1960	264	95	14
1970	304	108	19
1980	313	119	22
1990	285	126	27

*Unrestricted principals

Source: Office of Health Economics 1992

provision of general practitioner services available for people in their last year of life has increased in quantitative terms since 1969.

A further change since 1969 has been a decline in home visiting by general practitioners. Statistics from the General Household Survey (which only goes as far back as 1972) are given in Table 1.4. The decline has been partly brought about by increases in telephone consultations, but for the elderly has also involved an increasing proportion of consultations on surgery premises. This has particular implications for people who may have difficulty with mobility, as many elderly people do, and one of the important purposes of this book will be to assess how this change, as well as others in general practice, has affected those in the last year of life.

Table 1.4
Percentage of NHS general practitioner consultations by site (Great Britain)

Year	Surgery		Home	
	All ages	75+	All ages	75+
1972	73	36	22	61
1980	78	46	15	49
1989	78	47	15	49

Source: OPCS 1975, 1982, 1991.

Table 1.5
Changes in the district nursing service: 1972-87/8 (England)

Year	District nurses (wte) per 1000 population aged 65+	Persons aged 65+ treated (rate per 1000)
1972	656.1	133.3
1980	503.2	202.6
1987/8	492.2	220.7

Source: DHSS 1982, DoH 1990

Changes in domiciliary services

The demographic changes described earlier mean greater demands being placed on care in the community. Although the vast majority of this is provided informally by family and friends, a substantial proportion is provided by district nurses, home helps and other health or social services such as chiropody and meals on wheels. Some indication of changes in the community nursing service is given in Table 1.5. (The table only goes back to 1972 since figures before that are not comparable due to changes in the designation of nurses). The table shows that while the proportion of nurses for every 1000 people aged 65 or more in the population has declined, the proportion of people aged 65 or more who were treated by such a nurse has risen. It is unlikely that the increase in treatment has been gained entirely by providing less for other age groups, though this may be a part of the explanation. What is more likely is that the amount of time given by each nurse to each patient has declined, although this is not recorded in official statistics. What effects will this have had on the quality of the service, and has it affected those in their last year of life?

Other important domiciliary services are meals on wheels, home help and chiropody which, as Table 1.6 shows, have all shown quantitative increases in the period between 1969 and 1987. What the statistics do not reveal, however, is whether the increase is in line with need. The study reported in this book aims to answer these and other such questions.

Table 1.6
Meals, home helps and chiropody: 1969-87 (England)

Year	Meals provided in recipients' homes (millions)	Home helps per 1000 population 65+	Chiropody: persons treated 65+ per 1000 population 65+
1969	13.2	5.1*	132*
1980	27.0	6.9	188
1987	32.0	8.0	234

*England and Wales

Source: DHSS 1977, 1978, 1982, DoH 1990

Changes in institutional provision

Since 1969 death has increasingly become an event that occurs in hospital. In 1969 56% of deaths in England and Wales occurred in hospitals, with 35% occurring in peoples' own homes (Registrar General 1969). By 1987 the proportion of hospital deaths had risen to 64%, and the proportion of deaths in peoples' own homes had fallen to 25% (OPCS 1987). Although this might suggest that hospitals have become increasingly important in the care of the dying, other trends indicate otherwise. The average length of stay in NHS hospitals in England and Wales halved during the same period, from 26 days to 13 (Office of Health Economics 1992). These statistics suggest that hospitals in 1987 may play a rather different role in the care of those in their last year of life than in 1969, with perhaps more but shorter admissions, particularly near the time of death.

Another change for older people has been the proportion living in residential homes, as is shown in Table 1.7. As well as an overall increase in the proportion residing in such homes, the nature of this provision has changed, with a far higher proportion in 1987 being privately run. An important purpose of this book is to describe the impact of these changes in institutional care upon those in their last year of life.

Table 1.7
People aged 65+ in residential homes 1969-87

Year	Number of people aged 65+			Rate per 1000 people aged 65+
	Local authority	Voluntary	Private	All homes
1969*	89,975	23,239	17,369	20.7
1987[a]	99,750	25,105	84,946	28.3

*England and Wales
[a]England

Source: DHSS 1982, DoH 1990

Hospice care

The hospice approach, which is largely concerned with terminal cancer care, emphasises the relief of distressing symptoms, particularly pain (Twycross 1978), in preference to "heroic" attempts at cure that may be at the expense of patients' quality of life. Hospice staff also generally try to avoid a "conspiracy of silence" about death, whereby people who are medically recognised to be dying have this knowledge kept from them, a situation which is seen as abandoning the patient to his or her fears. Cicely Saunders' concept of "total pain" (Saunders 1978) which is addressed by hospice care involves a unified view of the distress of dying and of appropriate care, with physical, mental and spiritual dimensions of suffering all being the concern of the hospice team.

In addition, hospice care is characterised by a willingness to support carers at home, using hospice beds for respite or crisis care. Thus specialist domiciliary nursing teams with an advisory and supportive role are widespread (see Table 1.1). This goes with a general involvement with patients' families, involving the support of family members after as well as before a death.

At one level, hospice care may be understood as a part of a general reaction against the excessive medicalisation of areas of life (such as childbirth) that many considered to be "natural" that has characterised the public mood from the 1970s onwards. Seen most recently in the establishment of the Natural Death Centre, to parallel the earlier Natural Childbirth movement (Albery et al. 1993), this mood encompasses distrust of professional authority and an attempt to return to what are thought to be the values of older traditions.

Yet at the same time the development of a new medical expertise in the growing speciality of palliative medicine warns us against viewing the movement as solely a "grassroots" community movement. This may indeed be a more accurate characterisation of hospices in the USA (Abel 1986). James and Field (1992) have reviewed the growth of the hospice movement in the UK, suggesting that from being in its early days in radical opposition to mainstream health care, the hospice approach has now become institutionalised as a specialty within the main health care system. The effect of these trends, if they have occurred, on the actual delivery of care remains to be explored. It is at least possible, as is suggested by Parkes' study of standards of pain control in St Christopher's and surrounding hospitals (Parkes and Parkes 1984) that standards of care in the "mainstream" have been catching up with those in the hospice movement.

The study reported in this book enables some assessment of the impact of the hospice movement in the period between 1969 and 1987 on the care of people who die. Matters such as the numbers served by hospices (which are not recorded in official statistics), a comparison of people who receive hospice services with others, and general reflections on the role of this specialist terminal cancer care service are reported. Because the study draws on a random, representative national sample of deaths the contribution of hospices is placed in the context of life before death in general, and is not just confined to discussion of death from cancer or AIDs as is so much of the literature concerning the experience of dying.

Awareness of death

Hospice care can be viewed as a reflection of much broader changes in attitudes towards death and dying that have been gathering pace since the 1950s, characterised by an increased academic, professional and public awareness of death. The publication of Geoffrey Gorer's essay "The pornography of death" in 1955, according to Prior (1989), "seemed to presage an opening of the flood gates as far as publications on the subject of "Death" were concerned." Amongst the flood of books and articles, some of the better known are Gorer's subsequent book on *Death, Grief and Mourning* (1965), Herman Feifel's *The Meaning of Death* (1959), Glaser and Strauss on *Awareness of Dying* (1965), Elisabeth Kubler-Ross *On Death and Dying* (1970), Phillippe Aries' *The Hour of our Death* (1981) and Norbert Elias' *The Loneliness of the Dying* (1985).

These, and a host of other pieces written by health care practitioners, psychologists and sociologists have contributed to a perception that a "denial of death" has been characteristic of Western societies. Gorer took the view that in English society there was an absence of adequate mourning ritual to help people in grieving their dead. Kubler-Ross argued that dying had been taken over by impersonal technological and bureaucratic routines, and devoted her energies to discussing impending death with the terminally ill. The feeling that the dying were isolated, ignored by modern medicine and shunned out of fear and embarrassment by those around them is expressed by Aries. Glaser and Strauss analyse the interactions in hospital wards that lead to "closed awareness," where a conspiracy of silence keeps knowledge of their impending deaths from dying people. Norbert Elias sums up some of the central feelings of those involved in this opening up of awareness about death:

> Closely bound up, in our day, with the greatest possible exclusion of death and dying from social life, and with the screening-off of dying people from others... is a peculiar embarrassment felt by the living in

the presence of dying people. They often do not know what to say...
Feelings of embarrassment hold words back. For the dying this can be
a bitter experience... It is not always easy to show to people on their
way to death that they have not lost their meaning for other people...
If this happens, if a person must feel while dying that, though still alive,
he or she has scarcely any significance for other people, that person is
truly alone. (Elias 1985).

At the same time there has been an increased awareness of the limitations of institutional care across a variety of settings, perhaps the best known of these being Goffman's assessment of *Asylums* (Goffman 1961). This critique, too, has been reflected in the literature on death and dying. As well as Glaser and Strauss's documentation of hospital routines surrounding the dying, Sudnow's (1967) study of "social death" in hospitals was influential in inspiring moves to create more caring and humane institutional environments for the dying.

The hospice movement, then, can be located within these broader changes of attitude towards the dying. It is a specific response to the feeling that the dying should be accompanied by those around them as they approach their end. It might be expected that these changes in social attitudes might have influenced people outside the hospice movement as well, and that this could be reflected in the experiences of dying people in a variety of settings.

Life before death in 1969

In 1973 *Life before Death* (Cartwright, Hockey and Anderson) was published, describing a study of the last year of life of 785 people who had died in 1969, based on interviews with their relatives, friends and others who knew the people when alive. The idea for this study (as described in Cartwright and Seale 1990) had arisen opportunistically on the basis of the availability of a suitable sampling frame. Having recently carried out a study of contraception based on a sample chosen from birth certificates (Cartwright 1970), Ann Cartwright turned her mind to the potential of death certificates. She reasoned that a study based on a random sample of adult deaths in England and Wales could give a picture of the way society cared for a group of people, many of whom would be old and most of whom would be sick, in the year before they died. Because people would not be identified by their needs for care - although clearly many of them would have great needs - the study would show the ways in which a multiplicity of services functioned, or failed to function.

The study revealed many inadequacies in services, problems of co-ordination between different types of services, failures of communication, and lack of practical, emotional and social support for the relatives and friends who bore the brunt of caring for the people who died. The conclusions emphasised the high level of unmet need - both in terms of domiciliary support such as home helps and district nurses, and in the adequacy of bed provision for the elderly in hospitals and other institutions. It also showed that the vast majority of care was provided by relatives and friends, a situation which contrasted "rather strangely" with the view of some doctors in the study who criticised relatives for not accepting reasonable responsibility for looking after family members at home.

In its recommendation that "there needs to be more emphasis in medical education on caring and relieving rather than curing," and its criticism of some doctors who were "apt to lose interest" in patients who were incurable, the study reflected the concerns of the then emerging hospice movement. It was widely read, and its findings supported those who were concerned to create better conditions for the dying.

The year before death in 1987

The 1987 study, funded by the Medical Research Council, was begun largely out of an interest in assessing the impact of the hospice movement on care of the dying. Its stated aims were as follows:

1 To describe the last year of the lives of a random sample of adults dying in 1987.

2 To make comparisons with the earlier study and identify changes in the nature and availability of care and in the attitudes and expectations of lay and professional carers.

3 To make some assessment of the influence of the hospice movement on these changes.

4 To describe, in more detail than was done in the 1969 study, the institutional care of people in the year preceding their death.

5 To determine the experiences and views of the doctors and nurses involved in the care of these people in the last year of their lives.

6 To describe the care and support given to close relatives both after and before the death.

Table 1.8
Study areas for "The year before death in 1987"

Area	Type	No. of deaths in 1986	Hospice services
Hyndburn and Rossendale	County	1927	None
Hart and Rushmoor	County	1232	None
Birmingham Central	Met.	2483	None
Kingston upon Hull	County	3055	Home care
Luton	County	1481	Home care
Rochdale	Met.	2436	Home care
Bromley (East)	Met.	1779	Home care
Lewes	County	1193	6.7*
Lambeth	Met.	2668	11.6*
Bradford (North)	Met.	2712	19.2*

*Hospice beds per 1,000 deaths.

The basic purpose of these descriptions, comparisons and assessments was to identify ways of improving the quality of life before death.

The new study aimed to repeat the methods of the earlier one, including sampling and much of the questionnaire design, so that comparability could be obtained. It would then be possible to identify trends over time. The methods of the 1987 are reported fully in a book which tells the detailed story of how the study was done (Cartwright and Seale 1990), but a brief summary is given here.

Sampling

The 1969 study was done in 12 randomly selected death registration districts in England and Wales, stratified first by county and London boroughs versus the rest, then by region. For a variety of reasons the 1987 study was based on a sample drawn from local authority areas, split into electoral wards. The areas were stratified first by the presence or absence of a hospice, and after that by region. This was to ensure that the sample was representative in relation to a key factor: the level of hospice services. As in 1969, 12 areas were randomly selected, but these were from England only, and were reduced to ten areas largely due to the refusal by two health authority ethical committees to allow the study to proceed. The areas thus included in the study are given in Table 1.8.

Eighty death certificates for people aged 15 and over registered in October and November 1987 were chosen in each area, making an initial sample of 800 deaths. In addition (and reported in this book only in the sections where hospice care is considered) a further 11 deaths in hospices were sampled.

Based on information on death certificates, interviewers went to the address of the person who died, or to that of the person who registered the death, and asked who might know most about the circumstances of the person who died. The person thus chosen for interview was asked for the names and addresses of the deceased's general practitioner and for information which would make it possible to identify the hospital consultants, hospices and domiciliary nurses who had been involved in the last year of life.

A postal questionnaire asking for general practitioners', consultants' and domiciliary nurses' general views on care of the dying was then sent. In addition, interviews about the care of specific people in the sample were sought with consultants and domiciliary nurses.

Response rate and representativeness

Most of the initial interviews with relatives, friends and others were done between six and eight months after the deaths had occurred. In some cases the only person available for interview was an official, such as a care attendant in a residential home, or a coroner. Table 1.9 shows sample sizes and response rates for the various groups in the 1987 study.

Full details of the effect of non response are given in Cartwright and Seale (1990) but, to summarise here, comparisons with national statistics revealed no major biases in the response to the main study on matters such as place or cause of death. There was a slight over representation of deaths among people aged 45-54 which was attributable to the loss of two study areas. Failure to interview someone about all the sample of deaths in the remaining areas resulted in some bias between areas and possibly an under representation of those who lived alone and were not married.

The relationships of the people who were interviewed in the first phase of the study to those who died are shown in Table 1.10 for both the 1969 and 1987 studies.

Table 1.9
Sample sizes and response rates: 1987 study

Survey of:	Sample size	Response (N)
Relatives, friends and others in the community (the "main study")	800	80% (639)
(With 11 extra hospice deaths)	811	80% (646)
General practitioners	397	62% (245)
Consultants		
General	323	65% (211)
Specific episodes	525	43% (226)
Domiciliary nurses*		
General	100	92% (92)
Specific	125	90% (113)

*The apparently high response rate for domiciliary nurses masks the fact that it was only possible to identify a nurse in 45 per cent of all episodes of care reported by relatives, friends and others.

The majority of people seen on both studies were close relatives but more of those on the 1987 study than in 1969 were officials - usually staff in residential homes.[1] This reflects the increase in people living and dying in such places. When sons and daughters are taken together with sons and daughters in law there is a decline in the proportion of these responders from 1969 to 1987 (from 37 per cent to 29 per cent), reflecting their increased mobility as well as the likelihood of their parents living in homes and a decline in family size.

People less close to the deceased who, presumably, knew less about the person's affairs, were less likely to be able to name a general practitioner. Among the general practitioners who were identified the main biases in their response rates related not to the characteristics and circumstances of the patients but to attributes of the doctors themselves. Younger doctors, those trained in Britain, those in larger partnerships and trainers were more likely to reply.

It was more easy to identify district nurses than other types of domiciliary nurse, so the replies are therefore biassed towards this type of nurse. People who died at home and those dying from cancer were over represented in the responses from nurses as were those receiving more care. The response from consultants was skewed in a number of important respects, there being a tendency for cancer patients, episodes of terminal care or care resulting in death, and hospice episodes to be over represented.

Table 1.10
Respondent's relationship to the person who died

	1969 %	1987 %
Husband/wife	39	36
Son/daughter	30	26
Son-in-law/daughter-in-law	7	3
Brother/sister including in-laws	8	6
Other relatives	6	8
Friend or neighbour	7	10
Staff of residential home	3	10
Coroner or other official	-	1
Number of deaths (=100%)	785	639

The structure of this book

This book is based on articles that were printed in a variety of academic journals between 1989 and 1993. A decision was taken early in the study to report the results as a series of papers, targeted on particular professional audiences. It was felt that this was the best means of disseminating results to those who were in a position to act upon them. Having written and published some 17 articles, however, it became clear that there was an audience who would welcome the collection of all the results from the study under a single cover; hence this book.

The text is divided into four parts, each with an introductory section. In Part I, some of the key changes between 1969 and 1987 are summarised so that readers may gain an initial overview of trends over time (chapter two). Part II concerns the experience of illness, death and bereavement, focusing initially on the communication issues and awareness of dying (chapter three), followed by a chapter on the role of religion in peoples' lives as they approach death (chapter four). The experience of caring for dependent and dying people is then described (chapter five) and this is followed by a discussion of the influence of social class on peoples' experience of illness and care (chapter six). Part II ends with a chapter on the particular situation of those who die when they are very old (chapter seven).

Part III concerns hospice, hospital and other forms of institutional care. The central role of the hospice movement in reflecting and influencing the transformation of the public debate about dying has been referred to already. This part of the book shows how hospice care is experienced by those who receive it (chapter eight), and then places this form of care in the context of dying in general (chapter nine). Peoples' experiences of hospitals (chapter ten), residential and nursing homes (chapter eleven) as well as day centres (chapter twelve) are then discussed. It will become evident that these forms of provision serve many more people in the last year of life than do hospices, and the argument that thinking about the care of the dying should increasingly consider the role of these forms of institutional care is considered.

Part IV considers in more detail than other parts of the book the views of the health care professionals who were surveyed, concerning issues of care in the community, particularly the issue of whether the right balance between community and institutional care is achieved (chapter thirteen). This part of the book then moves on to consider specifically the role of general practitioners (chapter fourteen) and community nurses (chapter fifteen), as well as the experience of these services by dying people, their relatives and friends. In chapter sixteen relationships and communication between the different professionals involved in care are discussed.

The book ends with a concluding chapter (chapter seventeen) that draws out the more important findings, and discusses prospects for the future.

Notes

1. Throughout this book either tests of differences in proportions or chi square tests have been applied to the data constantly and have influenced decisions about what differences to present and how much verbal "weight" to attach to them. Attention is only drawn to differences which are unlikely to have occurred by chance five or more times in 100 unless specifically stated.

2 Changes since 1969

This chapter reports on the differences and on the similarities between the 1969 and 1987 studies and shows how the many changes in the intervening years affected the lives of people in the twelve months before they died. It looks at the symptoms reported for the people who died, at the help and care they had been given by hospitals, other residential institutions, general practitioners and community nurses. Respondents were also asked about their own and the deceased's person's knowledge of the diagnosis and prognosis and about the deceased's social circumstances.

Age, circumstances and place of death

The proportion of deaths occurring at age 75 or more was 54 per cent in 1987, an increase from the 1969 proportion of 40 per cent. However in the 1969 study the sample contained an excess of cancer deaths and a related deficit of deaths of people aged 75 or more. Partly because of this bias a number of the comparisons between the two studies are made between cancer deaths and others. National statistics give the proportion of deaths to people aged 75 or more as 45 per cent in 1969, still less than the proportion observed in 1987. Table 2.1 gives further details of the age of the people who died in the two studies. The change was partly because of the rise in the proportion of adults in the population in this age group but, as indicated in the introductory chapter, there was also an increase in the expectation of life during this time.

In both 1969 and 1987 one in ten of the deaths were unexpected with no previous illness or warning (the 1969 definition) or sudden deaths with no illness or warning or time for care (1987 definition). These were mainly deaths due to ischaemic heart disease or accidents.

Table 2.1
Age at death and place of death in 1969 and 1987 samples

Age at death	1969 %	1987 %
15-44	5	4
45-64	25	19
65-74	30	23
75-84	27	31
85+	13	23
Place of death		
Hospital	46	50
Hospice	-	4
Other institution	5	14
Own home	42	24
Elsewhere	7	8
Number of deaths (=100%)	785	639

Table 2.2
Household composition

	1969 %	1987 %
Lived alone	15	32
Lived with spouse only	32	38
Lived with spouse and other	20	14
Lived with other only	33	16
Number of deaths (=100%)*	670	508

*Excluding those in hospital or institution for a year or more before they died and sudden or unexpected deaths of those under 65.

The proportion dying in hospitals increased slightly between 1969 and 1987 (see Table 2.1), and whereas less than one per cent of those in the 1969 study died in a hospital or institution specialising in terminal care, this proportion had increased to four per cent in 1987. The largest increase was in the proportion dying in other institutions, mainly residential homes, while the proportion dying in their own homes fell markedly.

Where, and with whom living

Between 1969 and 1987 there was a rise from 9 per cent to 15 per cent in the proportion of people who had spent all the last year of their lives in a hospital or institution. Excluding these and also the sudden deaths of people under 65 the household composition of the people in the two studies are compared in Table 2.2. (The exclusions were made because the question about household composition was not asked for these groups on the later study). The proportion living on their own doubled while those living with people other than their husband or wife fell sharply. The proportion living with a spouse was similar for the two studies (52 per cent in both cases), but in 1987 fewer were living with others as well.

Hospital and other institutional care

The length of time people had spent in hospital or other institutions during the last 12 months is shown in Table 2.3. Fewer people in 1987 had not been in any institution during that year and more had spent the whole year in one.

Table 2.3
Length of time in hospital or other institutions in the year before death

	1969 %	1987 %
Not at all	30	16
Less than a week	12	15
One week but less than a month	21	23
One month but less than three months	19	21
Three months but less than six months	7	6
Six months but less than a year	2	4
A year or more	9	15
Number of deaths (=100%)	781	631

The other big change was in the number of admissions. In 1969 the average number of admissions to hospital during the last year of people's lives was 0.9; by 1987 this had increased by just over 50 per cent. The proportion dying in hospital had increased only marginally by comparison, so clearly there had been a substantial increase in the number of discharges from hospital to the community. Nevertheless, on both studies the majority of people, 89 per cent in 1969 falling to 81 per cent in 1987, spent most of the last year of their lives at home.

Table 2.4
General practitioner consultations in year before death

All consultations	1969 %	1987 %
0	4	6
1-4	22	32
5-9	20	21
10-19	25	22
20+	29	19
Home visits		
0	12	23
1-4	31	38
5-9	17	15
10-19	17	13
20+	23	11
Night calls (8pm - 8am)		
0	73	73
1	17	12
2-4	7	11
5+	3	4
Number of deaths excluding those who had been in hospital or institution for a year or more (=100%)	713	541

Care from general practitioners

Data from another, more general, study (Cartwright and Anderson 1981) show a decline in the amount of home visiting done by general practitioners, and this is reflected in the increase in the proportion of people who had no home visits from a general practitioner in the last year of their lives, and the fall in the proportion having 20 or more home visits (see Table 2.4). This cannot be attributed to a lower rate of home visiting among people living in residential homes (see chapter eleven). In addition there was a reduction in the proportion having 20 or more consultations, possibly because many people when they are old and ill are dependent on home visits and cannot get to the surgery (Cartwright 1990). The most frequent criticism of general practitioners on the 1987 study was of reluctance or failure to visit (see chapter fourteen), but this was not asked about in the 1969 study.

While general practitioners may have become less accessible to their immobile or housebound patients there was some indication that their communication skills had improved. Rather more of the respondents interviewed who knew the general practitioner of the person who died thought the doctor was easy to talk to in 1987 than in 1969 (87 per cent compared with 75 per cent) and that he or she had time to discuss things (82 per cent compared with 69 per cent). (If interviews with people other than relatives are excluded from these comparisons the differences between the two studies are reduced slightly but remain significant).

Care from nurses at home[1]

Similar proportions of the people who died in 1969 and 1987 (roughly a third) had been visited by a district nurse at home in the 12 months before they died. However, the length of time over which people were given this care had increased, with half those receiving care in 1987 having it for three months or more compared with just under a third in 1969. But the proportion receiving care on a daily basis was lower on the more recent study (41 per cent compared with 56 per cent). Jacoby (1990) reported nurse managers in the study areas who said that people had to be seen less frequently in order to meet increasing demands.

Care from home helps

This changed dramatically between the two studies. In 1969 10 per cent of people who died (excluding those in a residential home or hospital for the whole of the last year of their lives) had received some help from a home help. By 1987 this proportion had risen to 24 per cent. Nevertheless the proportion of people felt to be in need of such care or of more care had not

Table 2.5
Symptoms reported in 1969 and 1987 for cancer and other deaths

	Cancer deaths		Other deaths		All deaths	
	1969 %	1987 %	1969 %	1987 %	1969 %	1987 %
Pain	87	84	58	67*	66	72*
Trouble with breathing	47	47	44	49	45	49
Vomiting feeling sick	54	51	21	27*	30	33
Sleeplessness	69	51*	41	36	49	40*
Mental confusion	36	33	36	38	36	37
Depression	45	38	31	36	36	36
Loss of appetite	76	71	37	38	48	47
Constipation	42	47	23	32*	28	36*
Bedsores	24	28	13	14	16	18
Loss of bladder control	38	37	29	33	32	34
Loss of bowel control	37	25*	24	22	28	23*
Unpleasant smell	26	19	11	13	15	14
Number of deaths (=100%)[a]	215	168	570	471	785	639

*Difference between 1969 and 1987 significant at the 5% level.

[a]Small numbers of deaths for whom inadequate information was available are included in the total but have been excluded from this and other tables in this book when calculating percentages.

changed significantly: a further 13 per cent in 1969 and 14 per cent in 1987 were reckoned to have needed it while 44 per cent in 1969 and 33 per cent in 1987 of those having some help were thought to have needed more.

In both studies the home help services were concentrated among people of 65 or more who lived alone. In 1987 52 per cent of these had such help (35 per cent in 1969); even so 44 per cent of elderly people living alone in 1987 and not receiving this help were thought to need it.

Symptoms

The symptoms reported for people dying in 1969 and 1987 are shown in Table 2.5. The first thing that is striking is the similarity of the two sets of figures. Dying in 1987 was accompanied by the same sorts of symptoms as dying in 1969. That said, pain and constipation were reported for rather more people in 1987 than in 1969, sleeplessness and loss of bowel control for fewer. Deaths from cancer were associated with a high rate of several symptoms (see chapter nine) and the symptoms related to cancer and other deaths are also shown in Table 2.5.

The increase in pain and constipation was confined to people dying from causes other than cancer, and in addition there was an increase among this group in the proportion reported to have experienced vomiting or feeling sick. In contrast, among those dying of cancer in the two studies there was a fall in the proportion with sleeplessness and loss of bowel control.

There was an increase among those with mental confusion, depression and incontinence of bladder or bowel in the proportion who were reported to have had the symptom for a year or more: from 29 per cent to 55 per cent for mental confusion, 47 per cent to 60 per cent for depression and 25 per cent to 43 per cent for incontinence.

Awareness and information about death and illness[2]

Turning from the physical problems, care and circumstances of people dying in 1969 and 1987, what of their awareness of their diagnosis and prognosis? Has the more open discussion between patients and professionals (Lancet 1980) extended to the dying? To look at any changes those dying of cancer were considered separately from others as for cancer awareness of the diagnosis and prognosis are often linked and the likely outcome is often more certain. Indeed the questions asked about knowledge of diagnosis and prognosis are more clearly relevant to people dying of cancer than from many other conditions.

Between 1969 and 1987 there was a dramatic rise among people dying of cancer in the proportion thought to have known what was wrong with them and in the proportion who knew that they were dying. But there was no change among people dying from other causes. This can be seen in Table 2.6.

In 1969 those dying of cancer were thought to be less likely than those dying of other causes to know what was the matter with them. By 1987 the position was reversed: more of those dying from cancer than from other conditions were thought to have known the diagnosis. In 1987 more of those dying of cancer were thought to have known they were dying, whereas in 1969 there was no difference over this between the cancer and the non cancer deaths.

When respondents were asked to assess whether they thought it was best that the person knew or did not know that they were likely to die or whether it would have been better if they had or had not known, there were no significant differences between the two studies in their assessments for those who knew, in spite of the big increase in this group for those people dying of cancer. Indeed, there were no significant differences in these assessments

Table 2.6
Dying person's knowledge of condition and prognosis

	Deaths from cancer		Deaths from other causes		All deaths	
	1969	1987	1969	1987	1969	1987
What was wrong	%	%	%	%	%	%
Knew	29	73	57	60	49	65
Did not know	49	16	27	28	34	24
Uncertain/Other comment	22	11	16	12	17	11
Number of deaths (=100%)	204	158	478	285	682	443
Likely to die	%	%	%	%	%	%
Knew certainly	16	44	18	22	18	30
Knew probably	21	20	20	20	20	20
Probably not	8	8	10	9	9	8
Definitely not	39	14	31	30	33	24
Unable to say	16	14	21	19	20	18
Number of deaths (=100%)	213	159	478	283	691	442

between the two studies when people thought to have known or not known and those dying of cancer or other causes are considered. But the proportion who felt it was "best as it was" was higher if the dying person was thought *not* to have known that he or she was likely to die. This was true in both 1969 and 1987. The figures are in Table 2.7. It also held for cancer deaths and for non cancer deaths. The overall proportion of respondents who felt the situation was "best as it was" showed a slight but significant decline for cancer deaths between 1969 and 1987.

In 1969 the respondents reported that they themselves were more often aware of the diagnosis and the prognosis than the person who died. This suggested that communications were restricted and the dying person treated as someone to be protected rather than informed. This was also so in 1987. The figures for diagnosis were 81 per cent of respondents knowing, 65 per cent of those who died, and for prognosis 60 per cent compared with 30 per cent. It also held for both cancer and non cancer deaths. An additional question which the general practitioners were asked in 1987 but not in 1969 indicates a possible reason for this: more of them said they were more likely to discuss a terminal prognosis with relatives (57 per cent) than with the patient (17 per cent). The rest made other comments.

Table 2.7
Proportion of respondents who felt the dying peoples' knowledge or lack of knowledge about the prognosis was "best as it was"

	Person thought to have:		All
	known	*not known*	deaths
Deaths from cancer			
1969	51% (79)	86% (84)	69% (163)
1987	51% (100)	76% (33)	57% (133)
Deaths from other causes			
1969	58% (168)	81% (188)	71% (356)
1987	64% (115)	80% (107)	72% (222)
All deaths			
1969	55% (247)	82% (282)	70% (519)
1987	58% (215)	79% (140)	66% (355)

Figures in parentheses are the numbers on which the percentages are based (=100%)

Conclusion

It is clear from these comparisons that there has been no dramatic move towards a prolongation of independent and symptom free life before death during the period between the two studies. The higher proportion of deaths occurring at 75 or more on the later study does not appear to have been accompanied by a greater number of symptoms in the last year of life but it seems to have resulted in longer periods of mental confusion, depression and incontinence for some. More people were spending the last year of their lives in institutions. For the others there had been an increase in short term hospital admissions, and more were living alone, fewer with people other than their husband or wife.

The rise in elderly people living alone or just with their husband or wife, together with the increase in hospital discharges led to greater need for supportive services at home, and there had been a substantial rise in the proportion who received home help care and some increase in the length of time people had help from district nursing services. But community services had not increased as much as the demand for them, and general practitioners became *less* accessible to people confined to their homes in the last year of their lives. The people who died had fewer home visits in 1987 than in 1969 and a fifth of the respondents were critical of this aspect of the general practitioner's care.

If our respondents were right, many more of those dying of cancer in 1987 than in 1969 were aware of this. But the proportion of respondents who felt the dying person's knowledge or lack of it was "best as it was" had not changed between 1969 and 1987 within the two groups - those who knew and those who did not. As more of the respondents felt it was best as it was when the dying person did not know they were likely to die than when they did, and as the proportion thought to know had increased for those dying of cancer, this means that altogether the proportion of respondents who felt it was "best as it was" had declined for cancer deaths between the two studies. Some respondents did not appear to appreciate the increase in openness between the two studies. Where does this leave the policy of more open communication? The answer must be uncertain. This is one issue over which it would be particularly relevant to have the views of the people who died. We cannot tell whether respondents were right in their assessments of what was best for their dying relative. It may be that some of the people who were dying felt excluded from the communications between doctors who were caring for them and their relatives, and they could have felt angry, lonely or frightened as a result. It may be that doctors and relatives collude to protect themselves from embarrassment and anxiety. If doctors more often talked to patients rather than their relatives first the different pattern of awareness among patients and relatives might change and with it the feelings of all three groups. The situation could also change if doctors had more training in communication with dying patients (56 per cent of the general practitioners in 1987 said they would like this and 33 per cent said they found it "rather difficult" or "difficult" to cope with their own emotional reactions to death and dying - see chapter fourteen).

Another question unanswered by these studies is the extent to which the trend towards more open communication can be attributed to the hospice movement. Certainly it appears to be confined to those dying of cancer and at present hospice care is almost exclusively confined to people with cancer. In the 1987 study hospice patients were more likely to know they were dying (see chapter eight) than other people dying of cancer, but the difference between the 1969 and 1987 studies remains when hospice patients were excluded from the later study.

It is possible that other observed changes which were also confined to those dying of cancer (the decline in sleeplessness and loss of bowel control) may be associated with improvements in care initiated by the hospice movement. That there was an increase in some other symptoms (pain, vomiting and constipation) among those dying from other causes, suggests that these people might benefit from greater skills and attention.

In 1987 as in 1969 dying was often an unpleasant and painful process. There remain many inadequacies in our services to alleviate the distress and create a comforting and supportive environment for the final event in our lives. Technical skills may have contributed to the prolongation of lives, but adequate services are needed to ensure that this extension is not sometimes a misery for both people who die and their relatives.

Notes

1. Sudden or unexpected deaths and those for people in hospital or other institutions for all the last year of their lives have been excluded from this section to make the data from the two studies comparable.

2. In this section those under 65 who died unexpectedly or suddenly have been excluded and information from respondents who were not relatives or close friends has also been excluded. In addition in 1987 a further 34 nearly sudden deaths of people with no previous illness or incapacity have also been omitted as these questions were not asked about them. This latter group cannot be identified in the 1969 study.

Part I
THE EXPERIENCE OF ILLNESS, DEATH AND BEREAVEMENT

Part I

Introduction

As described in the previous two chapters, an important change in social attitudes since the 1950s appears to be a greater willingness to talk about death. This is associated with a professional view that being more open with patients about serious medical conditions, and about the likelihood of dying, is desirable in terminal care. This is, in large part, a change that has been influenced by the psychological sciences, in which there is an emphasis on the therapeutic value of talking through fears and worries so that they may be more effectively managed.

Some writers (for example: Rose 1989) have seen the growth in psychotherapeutic influence in the twentieth century as an extension of surveillance. This involves the view that increasingly numerous aspects of life have been subjected to professional expertise, attempting to guide people towards fulfilment and happiness under the watchful gaze of a host of psychologically informed personnel - therapists, child guidance workers, health visitors, counsellors, social workers and doctors. In relation to the dying, Armstrong (1987) has described the approach to communication promoted by Kubler-Ross (1970 - see chapter one) as a modern form of confession, and relates this to a decline in religious authority: "innocent and guilty alike (have) the truth exacted and the confession heard." (Armstrong 1987).

The view that psychotherapy is analogous to a confession rather than a willing acknowledgement of personal distress is perhaps far fetched, but the debate alerts us to the tension between older forms of authority based in religion, and their secular replacements. The first two chapters in this section of the book show how dying people experience the rival discourses of psychology and religious belief. In chapter three the attitudes towards communication of the doctors and nurses involved in the care of the people who died are described. We then compare this with what happened in practice, using the reports of relatives and friends concerning communication about diagnosis and prognosis. The role of religious faith in peoples' preparation for their deaths is then explored in chapter four, together with the role of religion in the lives of respondents, who were often struggling with feelings of loss and bereavement at the time of the interview.

In chapter five the experience of relatives and friends who cared for those who died is discussed in more detail. Here, the effect of demographic changes on the availability of informal care is explored from the perspective of those providing such care. The extent of informal care, and the stress involved when the burden is great and the carers themselves are perhaps elderly or have difficulties related to their health, is described.

Much concern about the loneliness of dying (Elias 1985), and about the benefit for relatives of being able to say goodbye to those who die (Cathcart 1988), centres on whether those close to the dying person are present near the time of death. A death at home appears to many to offer more opportunity for such leave taking than dying in an institution. Support for the bereaved, as well as support for the dying, has become a topic of psychologically informed professional interest (Worden 1991). Views about the place of death, events close to the death itself, and the degree of support experienced by relatives - either from professional or informal sources - are described in chapter five.

The dominance of accounts at the psychological level in the literature on dying is perhaps understandable. Contemplation of death and bereavement reminds us of our own mortality and potential for loss, and informed attempts by psychiatrists such as Parkes (1972) or Hinton (1967) can be helpful in making sense of our feelings about this. Less obviously, our experience of old age and dying is influenced by more than personal psychology alone. Sociological variables determine much in our lives, and the effect of social class on the experience of illness and health care is perhaps the best documented of such variables. Chapter six reports the influence of social class on the experiences of the people in the study, and assesses the proposition that there may have been changes in social class inequalities during the period between the two studies.

Age is another key variable that determines the experience of health and of care. However, as noted in the introductory chapter of this book, there is something of a separation between professionals concerned with terminal cancer care and those concerned with the care of the elderly. This is reflected in the separate disciplines of palliative medicine and gerontology, in the distinction that exists between hospice care and care in nursing and residential homes, and in separate structures of professional training and advancement.

In chapter seven we attempt to contribute to a greater understanding of the issues that arise in dying when very old. The chapter reports the social and demographic circumstances of people in the sample who died aged 85 or more, compared with those of younger people, and highlights the particular situation of women and those who live alone. The degree to which the very old have needs for care that are different from younger people, and the extent to which these are met by the different services available is discussed.

The chapters in this section demonstrate the value of a study of a representative sample of deaths. Because the full variety of circumstances in which people die is included it is possible to gain a much broader picture than is provided in much of the existing literature on dying. The relevance of an approach to dying largely derived from the experience of terminal cancer care is put into perspective. Because the sample was not dependent on records of service use the extent to which formal services reach the community and address needs appropriately can be assessed. These chapters also help in understanding at a personal level what we might expect as we approach our own deaths.

3 Communication and awareness

In the medical literature a great deal has been written about what and how to tell the terminally ill about their condition, reflecting a move towards openness in what is advocated for and by doctors over the past 30 years. Novack et al. (1979) replicated a study done by Oken (1961) on United States physicians' preferences about telling cancer patients their diagnosis and found a marked change of policy, with 98 per cent of the later sample saying they usually told the patient, whereas 88 per cent in 1961 usually did not tell. In Britain the shift may be judged by the following two quotations by authors discussing what to tell the terminally ill:

> If patients do ask, it is always well to be guarded and to keep up hope; these days patients hear so much of the wonders of science that they feel something might be done, and it is always well to evade a definite answer. The answer should always be left to someone of responsibility, preferably the doctor or the matron...in a ward it can best be done at night when other patients are asleep. (Hughes 1960).

> In the past twenty years doctors have become more inclined to tell patients with cancer the truth about the diagnosis..(this change) is here to stay and we should start to train our students so that they will be able to help their patients without some of the anxieties still experienced by an older generation of doctors. (Lancet 1980).

The growing hospice movement may have been responsible for much of the change in attitudes, as openness about illness and death is a key element of the hospice approach. There is an increasing interest in training courses that help professionals develop their counselling skills in this area (Maguire and Faulkner 1988). However, data on what happens in practice, and on trends over time, are patchy in Britain. A number of studies (for example: Bowling and Cartwright 1982, Hinton 1963, McIntosh 1977, Rees 1972, Ward 1974, Wilkes 1965) have reported on what terminally ill people in Britain know about their condition, but samples have been drawn in different ways making comparability difficult and trends over time hard to establish. Moreover, it is likely that the communication issues in cancer (the focus of most studies in this area) are rather different for those with other conditions.

In this chapter we first describe the attitudes and intentions, expressed by doctors and nurses who were interviewed, about communication issues. This is compared with what happened in practice according to relatives and friends. The results show the proportion of people said to have known what was wrong with them and that they were likely to die. The results also show who told them, if anyone, and what their reactions were to the news and to the way in which they were told. Situations of "closed awareness" (Glaser and Strauss 1965) in which the truth was kept from the dying person by relatives, are identified.

The general views of doctors and community nurses

Hospital doctors, general practitioners and community nurses, in total 548, were asked whether they found it easier, in caring for people who were dying, if the person was aware that they were dying or unaware. Most (81 per cent) said they preferred awareness, with nine per cent saying they preferred patients to be unaware and 10 per cent making some other comment. No significant difference between the three groups was found.

All three groups were also asked how easy or difficult they found it to deal with their own emotional reactions to death and dying. Excluding the four per cent of respondents who were unable to answer in these terms, the majority (70 per cent) said they found it easy or fairly easy, the rest saying they found it difficult or rather difficult. The 211 hospital doctors were more likely than either of the other two groups to say they found it easy or fairly easy (78 per cent as opposed to 66 per cent of the 245 general practitioners and 61 per cent of the 92 nurses).

An open question on all three questionnaires asked whether the doctor or nurse had any general guidelines, views or philosophy about what, if anything, to tell patients when they were dying. Fourteen per cent did not reply to this question, a further 6 per cent simply wrote that they had no general principles on this, and 16 per cent wrote that it depended on the individual, or that every circumstance was different. Of those that did reply with some general idea of how they approached this situation, most expressed a preference for truth or honesty, albeit tempered by various considerations. Only 15 of the 548 professionals said that they did not normally tell patients. Examples of this are: "Can always keep hope up. Don't tell them they are dying. Joke with them" (General practitioner); "We talk to the family and tell them the situation but unless the family request it I do not tell the patients. I say "you have an ulcer but we are treating it and we will do our best"" (Consultant geriatrician); "No, I play it by ear really. If they ask me I say "well let's talk to the doctor about it, see what he says." I avoid telling them too much" (District nurse).

Many of those who expressed a preference for telling patients the truth put this in an unqualified way. Thus they said "honest answers to their question"; "the truth"; "always be honest" and "respond with the truth". Many of these replies as in the first of these examples involved the notion of answering a patient's questions. This was sometimes developed by respondents so that it became clear that the patient's desire to know would have to be expressed before the truth would be given: "To be frank and honest with adequate respect to the patient's desire to know and requirements to know about his or her condition" (General practitioner); "Answer all questions truthfully" (General practitioner); "Offer as much clinical information as the patient is seeking and can cope with. (Consultant in the care of the elderly).

Answers that included these two themes of telling the truth, and doing so in response to patients' requests were the most common type of response. Many added qualifications or gave instances where they would or would not tell. Thus some mentioned how they treated relatives' wishes, sometimes in rather different ways: "Answer questions truthfully. Nearly always tell the whole truth. Patients' interests, not relatives', are paramount" (General practitioner); "I tell them the diagnosis only if they ask me. I never volunteer. On the other hand I have long discussions with relatives on all aspects of the problem of dying relations" (Consultant geriatrician).

The priority given to relatives by the doctors in the sample is shown by their answers to a question as to whether they were more likely to discuss a terminal prognosis with the patient or his or her relatives. Many (29 per cent) did not wish to answer in these terms, with most of these (26 per cent of the consultants for example) saying they would want to discuss such a matter with both. But of those that did make a choice, 75 per cent said that they were more likely to discuss the matter with relatives.

A number of themes common in other replies to the question about their general approach are illustrated in this reply from a consultant in general medicine: "Give them the opportunity to ask what they want. Answer their questions honestly, but don't thrust unasked for information on them. Never convey the impression that "nothing can be done" even if remission or cure is out of the question. Assurance that all will be done to relieve the various forms of distress."

In addition to the common wish to be honest in response to questions, this doctor suggests that some patients would not want to know and so should not have unasked for information forced upon them. Keeping up hope and reassuring patients about symptom relief were also common themes in the replies. In stressing that some patients would not wish to know all the facts, the right not to know was often pointed out as well as the need to take things slowly: "I tend to feel my way and tell the patients what they want to know. They will often tell me. I don't think you should confront them. I also don't think they always want to be told. You hold them and sometimes you don't need to put it in to words but to be ready to talk about it if they want to" (MacMillan Nurse). Reassurance, both generally and specifically, about symptom relief, was the aim of many respondents: "I promise adequate pain relief" (General practitioner); "Give them encouragement and let them know you support them" (General practitioner).

Some respondents mentioned the patient's religious or philosophical beliefs playing a part in what they chose to say: "Tailored according to philosophy of patient ranging form pragmatic biological approach to religious beliefs and after life" (Consultant cardiologist). Occasionally the doctor or nurse mentioned that his or her own religious beliefs played a part: "I believe there is a life after death and try to explain that death is only a temporary separation" (General practitioner). Only three respondents said, in answer to the question about their general approach, that they found it difficult to talk to patients about death, and these were all nurses. One said: "If they know their diagnosis it is easy to talk to them. If they don't I find it very difficult to talk to them" (District nurse).

General practitioners and hospital doctors were also asked to say whether they tended to encourage or avoid a situation with dying patients where the prognosis could be discussed. Such a question might be viewed as biassed in favour of the first option, but nevertheless 54 (12 per cent) of the doctors said they avoided such a situation. These doctors were more likely than others to not answer the question about their general approach or views (27 per cent of them as opposed to 15 per cent of others) or to say that they had no general approach or that it all depended on the individual (33 per cent compared with 19 per cent of others).

Field (1984) has presented evidence suggesting that nurses working in an environment where they feel free to answer patients' questions about death honestly, provide better quality care. This contrasts with situations where nurses are expected to refer such questions to doctors. The doctors in the present study were asked whether a nurse (a home nurse in the case of general practitioners, a ward sister in the case of consultants) should answer patients' question about whether they were dying, or refer them to the doctor. Nurses were also asked whether they would deal with such a question themselves or refer it to a doctor. Half the doctors said the nurse should answer the question herself, and 55 per cent of the nurses said they would do so. Thirty five per cent of the doctors would prefer the nurse to refer the patient to them, there being no difference between consultants and general practitioners on this. The nurses were less likely to say they would refer the patient to the doctor (22 per cent said this). It is likely that this represents a shift in perceptions of responsibility since 1969. A slightly different question was then asked of general practitioners and district nurses, but it included the option of referring a patient's request to his or her doctor. More nurses and doctors in 1969 expected the matter to be referred to a doctor: 31 per cent of district nurses and 49 per cent of general practitioners (22 per cent of all nurses and 38 per cent of general practitioners in 1987).

The general picture from these comments is that of professionals in this field preferring open communication with patients and their relatives. However, telling relatives first was the most common strategy advocated in both 1969 and 1987, and a substantial proportion of both doctors and nurses believed that nurses were not the appropriate people to discuss these matters. Respect for the wishes of those who did not want to know all the facts, and a gradual and supportive approach towards telling others is evident in the replies, and is in accord with the advice given by counsellors training professionals in this field (Maguire and Faulkner 1988). However, the question remains: What happens in practice?

What happened in practice

Who knows

People sometimes die suddenly, with no warning, and even after a long illness death can occur without being expected medically. Both of these situations were represented in the sample of deaths. Hospital doctors and community nurses, in their interviews about individual patients, were asked whether the death was expected, completely unexpected, or in between the two. The death was said to be expected in 68 per cent of the 226 episodes reported on by hospital doctors and 62 per cent of the 113 reported on by community nurses. Both types of professional reported more expected deaths from cancer than for other deaths (hospital doctors reported 88 per cent for cancer, 54 per cent for other deaths; nurses reported 70 per cent and 50 per cent). Equivalent data are not available for the 1969 sample, and while there is no reason to believe that the proportion of expected deaths might have differed significantly from 1987, this possibility should be considered in comparing the two samples for the proportions of people who knew they were dying.

As was shown in chapter two (Table 2.6) people in the 1987 sample were significantly more likely[1] than those in the 1969 sample to be said to have known both what was wrong with them and that they were likely to die. The results given in Table 2.6 also demonstrate that this difference was due to changes in what was known by those dying from cancer. Comparisons for those dying from cancer are significantly different between the two points in time for both knowledge of condition and prognosis. This was not the case for those dying from other conditions. In fact, the position in 1969 was such that people dying of cancer were less likely than others to be said to have known what was wrong with them; by 1987 this position was reversed, with a significant difference in the opposite direction. By 1987, those dying of cancer were significantly more likely than others to be said to know they were likely to die, a change from 1969 when there was no significant difference.

Table 3.1
Respondents' knowledge of condition and prognosis[1]

	Cancer deaths		Other deaths		All deaths	
	1969	1987	1969	1987	1969	1987
	%	%	%	%	%	%
What was wrong						
Knew	88	84	82	79	83	81
Half knew	4	9	8	8	7	8
Did not know	8	7	10	13	10	11
Number of deaths	202	159	465	281	667	440
Likely to die	%	%	%	%	%	%
Knew	77	79	67	50	73	60
Half knew	3	12	11	16	9	14
Did not know	20	9	22	34	18	26
Number of deaths	204	159	440	282	649	441

There were also differences in respondents' own knowledge, as is shown in Table 3.1, but these were not as dramatic as the differences for those who died. There were no significant differences for any of the groups concerning knowledge of condition, but respondents in 1987 were more likely to have known that the person was likely to die where the death was from cancer compared to deaths from other conditions. Comparison over time shows no change for the cancer group, but for those dying of other conditions a significantly lower proportion of respondents in 1987 compared to those in 1969 said they knew that death was likely.

It is possible that in cancer death is more likely to be medically expected, and that this explains why more of those dying from cancer in 1987, compared with those dying of other conditions, knew they were dying. However, the results from the professionals' accounts suggest otherwise. Hospital doctors and community nurses were asked, in cases where they said the death was expected, or "in between" being expected and unexpected, whether the patients and their relatives had known. Hospital doctors' reports confirm the picture for death from cancer: in 83 per cent of such hospital episodes involving cancer the patient was said by the doctor to know they were dying, whereas this was true in only 35 per cent of such episodes where cancer was not the cause of death. They reported that someone in the family knew the patient was dying in 99 per cent (all but one) of cases where the person died of cancer, but only 85 per cent of other deaths. For nurses, the differences were in the same direction as those for the doctors, but did not reach statistical significance. As medically unexpected deaths were excluded from the results from doctors and nurses, they suggest that people who were suffering from any recognisably terminal illness were more likely to know if the illness was cancer.

The increase in peoples' knowledge about their condition since 1969 may be encouraging for those who advocate a policy of openness, but it remained the case that in 1987 a substantial proportion of people knew less than did the professionals who cared for them. Just over a third of the people whose deaths were expected by hospital doctors and nurses were said not to have known they were dying. The doctors reported that in 34 per cent of the episodes involving an expected death the patient had not known; for nurses the figure was 28 per cent.

Glaser and Strauss (1965) have described in depth the painful situation of "closed awareness", where relatives keep from the dying person the knowledge that he or she is dying. The results from 1987 suggest that this may still be quite common. Respondents themselves knew what was wrong and that the person would die more frequently than the person who died: 81 per cent said they had known what was wrong, and 60 per cent said they knew the person would die (the figures for the people themselves, as stated

Table 3.2
Original respondents' and deceaseds' knowledge about whether the person would die[1]

		Respondent Knew	Half Knew	Did Not Know	All
	Yes certainly	31%	2%	2%	35%
Deceased	Yes probably	15%	6%	5%	26%
knew	Probably not	4%	2%	4%	10%
	No definitely	13%	3%	13%	29%
	All	63%	13%	24%	N=407 (100%)

earlier, were 65 per cent and 50 per cent). A comparison of respondents' and the deceased's knowledge is presented in Table 3.2 so that the nature of discrepancies between respondents' and the dying person's knowledge can be examined. The most common situation is one where both parties knew that death would be the outcome. But where there is a lack of congruence, it is more common that the person who died did not know they were dying, than the other way around.

Closed awareness was more common where the people who died were suffering from long term mental confusion, a condition that was less likely to affect those dying of cancer (see chapter nine). In cases where the respondent knew that the person would die, 50 per cent of people who suffered mental confusion for a year or more before death were said not to have known they were dying, compared to 21 per cent of others. The comment made by one of the consultants in the sample indicates how this may have happened:

> As a psychogeriatrician most of the patients dying in my long stay wards are demented patients. They would not understand they are dying. Therefore we mainly deal with the relatives and attend to their emotional needs. There are a few patients with other diagnostic variety. Circumstances permitting we would discuss the approaching end with these patients. This can happen only if they die a slow death from terminal illness such as cancer, but their understanding powers remain intact.

Who tells

The main reason why people suffering from terminal cancer in 1987 were more likely than in 1969 to know what was wrong and that they were likely to die was because someone had told them. This is shown by the data presented in Table 3.3. Hospital doctors were more likely in 1987 than in 1969 to tell these patients both their diagnosis and that they would die. In 1969 people who died of cancer who knew their diagnosis were more likely than those who did not die of cancer to have guessed it, but by 1987 this difference was no longer significant. Guessing that they were likely to die without being told was equally likely in 1969 and 1987 for people who did not die of cancer, but those who died of cancer who knew were significantly less likely to have had to guess this by 1987, and this, in turn, was due largely to a significant rise in the proportion of hospital doctors who told their patients. Hospital doctors were also more likely to tell non cancer patients their diagnosis in 1987, though not that they were likely to die. These results suggest that there has been a trend towards greater openness about diagnosis and death between doctors and patients, and this has been particularly marked in the case of hospital doctors and cancer patients.

Table 3.4 presents the same analysis for respondents' own knowledge, and a more mixed picture is apparent. More of those who knew that the person would die had guessed this without being told in 1987, and this was true for both types of condition. General practitioners were less likely to have given respondents information in 1987, and hospital doctors more likely although this did not reach statistical significance in the case of hospital doctors and respondents for those who died from cancer. These differences may reflect increased rates of hospitalisation, or a reliance on diagnostic practices increasingly the province of hospital doctors.

The difference in what the person who was dying and the respondent were told in 1987 is shown by the results in Table 3.5, which also demonstrate the relative unwillingness of professional to tell people that they were dying, and their preferences for telling relatives. The person who died was more likely to guess what was wrong and that they were dying, without being told than were respondents. Being told what was wrong was more common than being told that death would result for both sets of people. Professionals told what was wrong in more or less equal proportions to patients and respondents, but were more likely to tell respondents that death would be the result than they were to tell the person who was dying. General practitioners and hospital doctors did most of the telling, hospice professionals being involved hardly at all. Nurses were involved to a lesser extent than doctors and no nurses were involved in telling their patients that they were dying.

Table 3.3
People who knew what was wrong with them and that they would die: professionals who told them, by condition and year[a]

	What was wrong				Would die			
	1969		1987		1969		1987	
	Cancer	Non cancer	Cancer	Non cancer	Cancer	Non cancer	Cancer	Non cancer
	%	%	%	%	%	%	%	%
Who told:								
No one	40	18	23*	18	78	84	52*	85
General practitioner	25	61	28	56	5	11	12	9
Hospital doctor	31	17	50*	49*	9	4	28*	6
Hospital nurse	2	1	3	10*	0	0	0	0
Home nurse	0	0	1	3	0	0	0	1
Total number of people who knew (=100%)	52	268	115	191	74	161	94	127

*Significantly different from the same group in 1969 (p<0.05)

[a]Percentages may not add up to 100 per cent because in some instances more than one person told, and some were told by people other than those listed in the table (see Table 3.5)

Table 3.4
Respondents who knew what was wrong and that the person would die: professionals who told them by condition and year[a]

	What was wrong				Would die[b]			
	1969		1987		1969		1987	
	Cancer %	Non cancer %	Cancer %	Non cancer %	Cancer %	Non cancer %	Cancer %	Non cancer %
Who told:								
No one	3	9	2	12	4	17	13*	33*
General practitioner	49	60	30*	44*	44	53	26*	15*
Hospital doctor	46	19	56	37*	51	18	55	41*
Hospital nurse	5	9	10	9	6	12	6	13
District nurse	1	0	1	3	2	1	2	1
Total number of people who knew (=100%)	175	373	139	260	171	289	125	138

*Significantly different from the same group in 1969 ($p<0.05$)

[a]Percentages may not add up to 100 per cent because in some instances more than one person told, and some were told by people other than those listed in the table (see Table 3.5)

[b]Excludes respondents who were not relatives or close friends

The manner of telling

Where respondents were told that the person was likely to die from their disease, they were asked how it had happened and how they felt about the way they were told. Forty seven per cent praised the way they were told: "It was very sympathetic and very nice" (Daughter of a woman who died of a heart attack); "A bit of a shock at first - we didn't know why (the doctor) was coming. But it was well put over" (Son of a man who died of a stroke); "Doctor..... was very kind. We have to face these things" (Husband of a woman who died of cancer of the bowel). Another 47 per cent made comments that neither praised nor criticised the way they were told. Only 6 per cent were critical. For example:

Table 3.5
People who knew what was wrong and that death would result: who told the deceased and the original respondent (1987)*

	Told what was wrong		Told person would die	
	Deceased	Respondent	Deceased	Respondent
	%	%	%	%
No one	20	9	71	27
General practitioner	45	39	10	21
Hospital doctor	49	43	15	42
Hospital nurse	7	10	0	9
Hospice doctor	1	1	0	1
Hospice nurse	1	0	0	0
Home nurse	2	3	0	1
Original respondent	14	-	7	-
Deceased	-	14	-	5
Other person	8	-	2	-
Other professional	-	4	-	2
Other relative	-	6	-	4
Total number of people who knew (=100%)	306	399	221	302

*Percentages add up to more than 100 per cent because more than one person told in some instances.

> It was awful. We'd gone in to see her, my daughters and me, and the wife had first gone along the corridor to go to the toilet...and a nurse came out of the office and just said "You know your wife is dying don't you, and the doctor wants to see you tomorrow" and she went off. We were completely shattered. We had to hide in the corridor as my wife came back and went into her ward. We couldn't let her see us. We were in tears. Then I went to see the doctor the next morning and told him how the nurse had told us. He was cross about that and he was so good and explained all I wanted to know. (Husband whose wife died of breast cancer).

Respondents in cases where the person who died had been told by someone were asked how they felt about the way the person was told. Many of the people asked this question answered it inadequately, focusing on whether the person should have been told rather than how they were told. Of 26 who did answer the question, 11 praised the way it was done, 11 were neutral and four were critical. Examples of comments are: "The GP suggested it was a good idea to tell him, to which I agreed. I was so grateful. We could then talk quite openly and not have to hedge around it. He knew what he had to aim at. He was told nicely. I wasn't in the room" (Son of a man who died of cancer of the prostate); "Quite nice. He was told in a nice way because the doctor called him by his christian name. He would say, now George..." (Niece of an elderly man who died of bronchial pneumonia); "It was wrong in a crowded ward. They had broached it before, but when the results came through we were in the ward" (Daughter of a woman who died of lung cancer).

The respondents for people who had been told by someone were also asked how the person had responded. The most common response (17 out of 56, or 30 per cent) was that the person had accepted the news. For example: "She just accepted it and got on with arranging things. I think she felt she had had a long life" (Daughter of a woman who died of cancer of the liver).

Fifteen (27 per cent) said that the person had decided to fight the disease, a variant of this reaction being stoicism or denial. A typical example here is that of a woman who died of cancer of the bowel, whose husband said: "It made no difference. She could cope with it. She had a strong character and was courageous. She didn't cry, but pushed it to the back of her mind and said "what's for tea?"."

A number of respondents focused on the initial emotional reaction of the person, the most harrowing of which was a young man diagnosed with AIDS, whose mother said: "He became hysterical. He had a counsellor and a hospital doctor and several nurses there and they had to hold him down." However, an initial shock sometimes changed to something better. The niece of a man who died from cancer of the bronchus said:

> A month before his death we didn't want the doctors to tell him. We knew he would take it badly. The doctors said that if he asked they couldn't lie to him, but we didn't want them to tell him. He went to the GP and he told him the truth. But having said that he seemed to accept it so well. He obviously was terribly upset at first, crying a lot, but it was like a miracle. He had changed so dramatically. I felt that the doctors were right to tell him. He sorted everything out with his wife and he had a lovely death at the end.

When asked how accepting the person who died was of the fact that they were going to die 61 per cent of the people who knew they were likely to die were said to have been definitely accepting and 25 per cent fairly accepting. Eleven per cent were said to have been not at all accepting and 3 per cent made other comments.

Preferences about knowing

As shown in chapter two (Table 2.7) whether the person who died knew they were dying or not, most respondents (66 per cent) said they felt that things were best as they were. Of those people who were said to know they were dying, respondents in only 11 per cent of cases thought it would have been better not to have known, many more (58 per cent) saying that knowing had been best, the rest making some other comment. Of those who were said not to have known they were dying, respondents in only 3 per cent of cases felt it would have been better for the person to have known, 79 per cent saying that not knowing had been best, and the rest making some other comment. Speaking of their own knowledge of the person's death, only 3 per cent of respondents who knew the person was dying said they would have preferred not to know. However, of those who did not know, 30 per cent would have liked to know. This is a significantly lower proportion than in 1969 when the figure was 43 per cent.

Thirty seven per cent of respondents had themselves talked about the person's death with that person. Only one of the 90 people who had done this said that they were sorry to have done so, 90 per cent being glad. Of those who had not talked with the person in this way, 10 per cent wished they had, 65 per cent being glad they had not, the rest making some other comment.

Hospital doctors, where they were able to report on the patient's knowledge of prognosis, in all but one instance out of 93 said that the situation that prevailed was "best as it was". Nurses were similarly satisfied with how things were, with only three out of 67 saying that the situation was not "best as it was".

These results suggest general support for current practice, from both the relatives and friends of those who died and from professionals. In spite of the changes in practice that had occurred since 1969, the results in Table 2.7 show that respondents in 1987 were no more or less likely to feel that the level of knowledge that prevailed was "best as it was" except in the case of those who died of cancer where there was a slight but significant decline. In general, the move towards openness has been in line with the preferences of families and friends of the dying, albeit expressed retrospectively. On this topic, however, it may be that responses are influenced by a desire to perceive events in a favourable light. It is, of course, not possible to know the preferences of the dying people themselves.

Information and support received by respondents[1]

As was stressed by some of the professionals in outlining their approach to communication, providing information and support to the dying and their relatives is important. To find out whether this was given to original respondents, at least, they were asked in the first instance whether they were able to find out all they had wanted to know about the person's illness and how it was likely to affect him or her. Most (77 per cent) said they had found out enough, with 22 per cent saying they had not; a similar proportion as in 1969 when the proportion was 23 per cent. However, of those who said they had been told enough 8 per cent had wanted more explanation, and 6 per cent had not found out things as soon as they wanted. When those who said they wanted to know more were asked what it was they wanted to know more about, 71 per cent mentioned information about what was wrong with the person. For example: "When he went in with this by pass stroke, they would not tell us. My sister kept ringing up but they would not tell us what was wrong. Eventually she spoke to the doctor in the hospital and he said it was a stroke but he had got over it" (Son whose father died of a heart attack); "The results of the tests and X rays they had done, what they had found out, what was wrong with her, why they didn't help her" (Husband whose wife died of a heart attack); "How the cancer started, why, everything. I still don't know why" (Wife whose husband died of cancer of the tongue); "I knew he was losing weight rapidly so I felt I knew there was something the matter. I was not told anything. The doctor said it was trapped wind and I believed him. I wish someone had told me what was wrong. No one gave me any help. They seemed to skim over things and never tell me anything" (Wife of a man who died of lung cancer).

Thirty two per cent wanted to know more about the reasons for decisions taken by the doctors:"The choice they thought they were giving her with the second operation; why they did it" (Woman whose mother-in-law died of cancer); "The reason they could not give her pain killers by injection when they had to stop giving them orally because of her condition" (Son whose mother died of coronary thrombosis); "What the choices of treatment were. They never made it clear. They were always trying out different things to see if they worked" (Son of a man who died of stroke).

Fifteen per cent wanted information that would help them cope with the care that the person needed: "How to deal with it better. I know mental conditions are difficult but I think more understanding of the problem would have helped" (Wife who had looked after her husband with senile dementia for four years); "Once they knew it was cancer I would like to have known how it was going to affect her and how much care she was going to need....I did not know about how to do bed baths or having to turn her every two hours, or giving her all the drugs. They don't tell you about things like that" (Daughter whose mother died of liver cancer).

Respondents who felt they had not known enough about the illness were asked if they had asked anyone for this information. Forty four per cent of them had asked no one, slightly more than in 1969 when 40 per cent asked no one although this difference is not statistically significant. Of those who did ask someone, 56 per cent in 1987 asked a hospital doctor, 45 per cent a general practitioner and 38 per cent a hospital nurse. Forty one per cent had asked more than one person. In 1969 fewer had asked a hospital doctor (25 per cent).

Table 3.6 shows the people to whom respondents talked about the illness and what might happen. Sixteen per cent talked to no one. Relatives, nurses, the person who died and doctors were the most frequently mentioned with friends playing a lesser role. Doctors were found to be the most informative and relatives the most supportive. In 1969 general practitioners were more likely to be talked to by the respondent: 78 per cent in 1969 compared to 51 per cent in 1987. Hospital doctors were less likely to be talked to: 39 per cent compared to 56 per cent in 1987, as were hospital nurses (33 per cent compared to 44 per cent). Fifty four per cent of respondents in 1969 said the general practitioner had given them the most information and 23 per cent said the hospital doctors had done so, again showing that hospital doctors in 1987 were increasingly called on to give information, and general practitioners less so. This repeated finding probably reflects changed patterns of hospital admissions. Comparing the 1969 data with 1987, the average number of admissions to hospital in the last 12 months of life had increased by just over 50 per cent, and the proportion of deaths occurring in hospital or hospices rather than at home had also increased.

Conclusion

The results suggest that between 1969 and 1987 there was a move towards greater openness between doctors - particularly hospital doctors - and dying people and their families. More terminally ill people in 1987 knew what was wrong with them and that they were dying than in 1969, and the changed practices of doctors, particularly those in hospital, appear to be largely responsible for this. Although the hospice movement stresses the decision making role of nurses and probably fewer nurses in 1987 felt the need to refer to a doctor before answering patients' questions, nurses at the later date were not in fact more involved in "breaking the news". It may be that their involvement in communication is of a different nature. General practitioners' roles may have changed as well, from being the first person to break the news, to helping to support the person afterwards. These changes are also related to increased numbers of hospitalisations during the last year of life.

Table 3.6
Who respondent talked to about the deceased's illness and what might happen*

	Talked to	Gave most information	Found most helpful and supportive
	%	%	%
No one	16	-	-
General practitioner	51	29	14
Hospital doctor	56	34	12
Hospital nurse	44	14	12
Hospice doctor	3	0	2
Hospice nurse	4	0	0
Home nurse	19	5	5
Vicar, priest	9	0	1
Other professional	10	4	4
Person who died	44	6	5
Relative	72	6	37
Friend/neighbour	38	1	7
Anyone else	5	1	1
Total (=100%)	475	418	412

*Deaths of people with no apparent illness or incapacity have been excluded, as has information from respondents who were not relatives or close friends

Hospital doctors were more likely than others to say they found their emotional reactions to death and dying easy to deal with, prompting the speculation that emotional distance might make it easier for then to break the bad news. However, if this is the case, it does not seem to have resulted in them telling people in an insensitive manner. Few respondents had criticisms of the way they or the deceased were told. The occasional bad experience suggests that the cautiousness advocated by a large proportion of the professionals, namely waiting to be asked and taking things slowly is appropriate and appreciated. Indeed, in the majority of cases the situation that prevailed, whether of open or closed awareness, was felt by both the original respondents and the professionals, to be the best. Doctors, on the whole, appear to be succeeding in identifying those who want to know without violating the wishes of the minority of dying people and respondents who wish not to know. However, the retrospective nature of the accounts may have influenced the reporting of preferences in this area.

The results also suggest that it is in the case of those dying from cancer - the focus of the hospice movement - that much of the change has occurred. The prognosis is generally clearer in cancer than in other diseases likely to lead to death, and so the communication issues are somewhat different. Mental confusion also plays its part in what people can be told, and this is less common in cancer (see chapter nine). It is possible that better public knowledge about cancer could have caused the increase in the numbers knowing, but if this had been a major factor the relatives and friends of those who died of cancer would also have been more likely to know in 1987, but this was not the case. The change in what people dying of cancer are told has been radical and probably reflects the fact that attitudes about what people can be told about this disease and its likely outcome have changed.

Nevertheless, the results show that instances where the relatives are given information and the dying are not are still quite common. Dying people are still highly likely to be left to guess for themselves that they are dying, and the emotional isolation that this produces can only be guessed at in the absence of dying peoples' own stories.

Notes

1. Those under 65 who died suddenly or unexpectedly have been excluded from the comparisons in this section, as has information from respondents who were not relatives or close friends. In addition, in 1987 a few nearly sudden deaths with no previous illness or incapacity have been omitted.

4 Religious belief

In this chapter we attempt to answer the question of whether religious belief is a help around the time of death by looking at the reports of relatives and others about the religious faith of the people who died and the way they accepted their death, and at the religious beliefs of the close relatives themselves and the relationship of these beliefs to the way they coped with their bereavement.

According to a study by Davis and Jowell (1989) 34 per cent of British people said they had no religion. Conflicting results are reported from other studies about religion and fear of, or looking forward to, death. Two reported no meaningful relationship (Muchnik and Rosenheim 1982, Chaggaris and Lester 1989), two found religion to be helpful (Svenson 1961, Feifel and Branscomb 1973), and two showed a curvilinear relationship: those who were moderately religious reporting more anxiety than those who were either high or low in religiosity (McCardie 1981, Downey 1982).

The religious faith of the people who died

A third of the people who died were reported to have had a strong religious faith, half to have had some, and one in six not to have had any. (Eight per cent of our respondents could not answer this question and these people have been excluded from these proportions). When the person who died was said to have had any religious faith respondents were asked what faith or denomination the person belonged to. (The questions were asked in that order in an attempt to preclude a routine answer of "Church of England" for those not thought to have had any faith). The majority of those who died, 56 per cent, were said to have been Church of England, 12 per cent other protestants, 13 per cent Roman Catholics, 4 per cent to have a variety of other faiths and the rest not to have had any religious faith. A final question about the nature of people's beliefs asked whether they were thought to have believed in some sort of life after death. A third of the respondents said they did not know whether the person who died believed in some sort of life after death or not. Of the rest they thought that 66 per cent had believed in some sort of life after death, 20 per cent had not, and that 14 per cent were uncertain about this.

Those whose faith or denomination was described as Church of England were less likely than other faiths or denominations to be thought to have had a strong religious belief or to have a belief in some sort of life after death. Roman Catholics were the ones most often seen as having a strong religious belief, but they were no more likely than "other protestants" to believe in some life after death. The figures are in Table 4.1 which also shows that a sizeable proportion, a fifth, of those described as having no religious faith were thought to have believed in some sort of life after death.

Table 4.1
Variations with nature of faith or denomination

	Church of England	Other Protestant	Roman Catholic	Other	None
Proportion with a strong religious faith	26%	62%	76%	57%	-
Deceased thought to have believed in some sort of life after death	%	%	%	%	%
Yes	70	82	86	72	20
No	16	4	6	17	66
Deceased uncertain	14	14	8	11	14
Number of deaths (=100%)	305	65	68	23	84

Who has a religious faith?

Religious faith was perceived as more common among the old. More of those who died when they were under 65 were thought to have no religious faith: 26 per cent compared with 13 per cent of those dying when they were older; and 37 per cent of those aged 75 or more were described as having a strong religious faith compared with 28 per cent of those dying before they were 75. There was also a clear trend with age in the proportion thought to have believed in some sort of life after death, the older people who died were more likely to have believed in it, the younger less so (see Table 4.2)

Table 4.2
Age at death and belief in some sort of life after death

Deceased thought to have believed in some sort of life after death	Age at death				
	Under 55	55-64	65-74	75-84	85 or more
	%	%	%	%	%
Yes	52	57	63	69	74
No	30	30	25	17	13
Deceased uncertain	18	13	12	14	13
Number of deaths for which information available (=100%)	33	46	101	131	88

Another age variation, which is likely to have reduced the strength of the associations between age and beliefs, was that there were more Roman Catholics among those with any faith dying when they were relatively young, that is before 65: 24 per cent compared with 13 per cent of the older groups. There were also fewer "other protestants" in the younger group: 5 per cent compared with 16 per cent.

More women than men were thought to have a religious faith: 43 per cent of women compared with 22 per cent of men were described as having a strong religious faith while only 9 per cent of women compared with 23 per cent of men were thought to have none. There was no difference between the two sexes in the nature of their denomination or faith but more men were thought not to believe in any sort of life after death: 28 per cent compared with 14 per cent of the women.

Looking at housing tenure as an index of social class, more owner occupiers than council tenants were thought to have a strong religious faith, 38 per cent compared with 26 per cent, while more council tenants had none, 20 per cent compared with 13 per cent, but this last difference did not quite reach statistical significance. Similar proportions of the two groups were described as having some religious faith. Fewer of the owner occupiers than of the council tenants were Roman Catholics, 10 per cent compared with 19 per cent, more "other protestants", 18 per cent compared with 9 per cent, with similar proportions of the two groups being Church of England. Seventy per cent of the owner occupiers, 60 per cent of the council tenants were said to have believed in some sort of life after death - a difference which might occur by chance.

Did their religious faith help?

Respondents were asked whether they thought their religious faith had been a help to the person in the time before he or she died. They were unable to answer this for 32 per cent (this proportion was higher, 43 per cent, for those they felt had some religious faith than for those who had a strong faith, 13 per cent). Among the rest the proportion thought to have been helped was 63 per cent: 91 per cent of those with a strong faith but only 36 per cent of those with some. For 5 per cent of those with a strong faith it was thought to have been no help compared with 55 per cent of those with some faith. (They made other comments about 4 per cent and 9 per cent of the two groups). So among all the people who die for whom the information is available it would seem that roughly one in six had no religious faith, three fifths had a religious faith that was thought to have been helpful to them before they died and a quarter had at least some religious faith but it was not thought to have been helpful.

Altogether those belonging to the Church of England were thought to have derived less help from their faith than those in other faiths or denominations: 54 per cent compared with 78 per cent. But if the comparison is made holding the strength of their belief constant the difference disappears. Those whose religious faith was associated with a belief in some sort of life after death were also more often thought to have found their faith a help: 78 per cent compared with 12 per cent. There was no difference with age or housing tenure in the proportion with a religious belief who were thought to have been helped by it, but more women than men were perceived as finding it helpful, 70 per cent compared with 53 per cent. However, this last difference seemed to be attributable to the variation in the strengths of their beliefs.

Up to now the indicator of whether a belief was helpful has been simply whether respondents perceived a belief to be so, and therefore those without any belief have not been considered. But it is also possible to see whether those thought to have known they were dying were more likely to accept this if they had a religious faith. Respondents were asked whether they would describe the person as "definitely accepting, fairly accepting or not at all accepting." There was no difference in the reported religious beliefs of those thought to have known or not known that they were dying, but as Table 4.3 shows, acceptance of death was seen as more frequent among those with a strong religious belief. The difference between those with some belief and those with none might well have occurred by chance.

In addition, as Table 4.3 also shows, discussion of death between the respondent and the person who died was more likely if the person who died had a strong religious belief. Over this the difference between those with some, and those with no religious faith just fell short of statistical significance.

Table 4.3
Variations with religious faith in acceptance and discussion of death

	Strong	Some	None	All
Acceptance of death	%	%	%	%
Definitely accepting	80	56	46	61
Fairly accepting	16	26	36	25
Not accepting	4	13	11	11
Other comment	-	5	7	3
Respondent and deceased discussed death	%	%	%	%
Yes	57	31	15	37
No	41	67	73	59
Other comment	2	2	12	4
Number thought to have known they were dying (=100%)	85	116	35	257

While religious faith seemed to facilitate acceptance of death, belief in some sort of life after death did not. The proportions felt to be accepting of death were similar among those thought to believe in life after death and those thought not to do so. But acceptance was less common among those thought to be uncertain about whether or not there was a life after death: only 33 per cent compared with 66 per cent of those who believed there was some life after death, 64 per cent of those who did not. Uncertainty appears to mitigate against acceptance.

Over discussion of death with the respondent the ones who stood out were those believing in some sort of life after death, nearly half, 47 per cent of them were reported to have talked to the respondent about their death compared with a quarter of those who either did not think there was any sort of life after death or were uncertain about it. Discussion of death was much more commonly reported for those felt to be "definitely" accepting of their death: 55 per cent of them were said to have talked about it compared with 22 per cent of those described as "fairly" or "not at all" accepting.

Were the differences in acceptance and discussion of their death related to the characteristics of those with a religious faith? Sixty five per cent of women, 57 per cent of men were regarded as definitely accepting of their death and 43 per cent of women, 31 per cent of men had talked to the respondent about their death. Neither of these differences reached statistical significance. Similarly, 66 per cent of people dying when they were 75 or more, 55 per cent of those dying at a younger age were reported to be definitely accepting of their death - another difference which fell short of significance, as did the difference between those aged 85 or more when they died and the others in the proportion who had talked about their death with the respondent: 45 per cent compared with 35 per cent. There was one significant variation with housing tenure; more of the owner occupiers than of the Council tenants, had talked about their death to the respondent, 46 per cent compared with 27 per cent. All these observed "differences" were in an expected direction, but they are unlikely to account for all the marked relationship between people's religious faith and their reported reactions to their approaching death. But the faith of the respondents could contribute to their reports of the beliefs of the people who had died and how these had helped them.

The faith of relatives and close friends[1]

Similar proportions of the relatives and close friends (subsequently described as relatives) as of the deceased had a strong religious faith, some or none; the faith or denominations they belonged to were also similar. But fewer of the relatives believed in some sort of life after death, 52 per cent compared with 66 per cent of the people who died, and more of the relatives were uncertain about this, 25 per cent compared with 14 per cent. Similar proportions of the two groups did not believe there was some sort of life after death.

Table 4.4
Association between relatives' and deceaseds' religious faiths

	Relative's religious faith		
Deceased's reported religious faith	Strong %	Some %	None %
Strong	59	21	14
Some	34	69	41
None	7	10	45
Number of relatives (=100%)*	141	265	64

*Those who said they did know about the religious faith of the deceased have been excluded.

Table 4.5
Beliefs of relatives and deceased about some sort of life after death

	Relative believed in some sort of life after death		
Deceased thought to believe in some sort of life after death	Yes %	No %	Uncertain %
Yes	79	34	48
No	11	53	26
Deceased uncertain	10	12	26
Other comment	-	1	-
Number of relatives (=100%)	214	68	70

There was a strong, but by no means complete, association between the relatives' religious faith and those they reported for the deceased. This is shown in Table 4.4. There was also an association, shown in Table 4.5, between the beliefs of the two groups in some sort of life after death. But when the relative felt uncertain about this only a quarter of them thought that the deceased had shared this view.

The faith of the relative was related to their perception of whether the faith of the person who died had been a help to them if the deceased was described as having "some" rather than a strong religious faith. For these people their faith was thought to have been a help to 58 per cent when the relative had a strong religious faith, but only to 30 per cent when the relative had either some or no religious faith. (Relatives who were uncertain whether the faith of the person who died had helped them have been excluded from these comparisons). Whatever their own religious faith nine tenths of the relatives thought a strong religious faith had helped the person who died.

The religious faith of the relatives and friends did not vary significantly with their relationship (spouse, child etc.) to the person who died, neither did their belief in some sort of life after death. A relatively small proportion of the relatives who were aged under 55 said they had a strong religious belief, 24 per cent compared with 32 per cent of those aged 55 or more, but for them there was no association or trend with age in their belief about some sort of life after death. Nor was there any significant trend with age in the proportion describing themselves as Roman Catholics or as belonging to the Church of England, but among those with any faith 23 per cent of those under 45 compared with only 4 per cent of older relatives said they belonged to religions other than Roman Catholic, Church of England or other protestant. Again women more often than men said they had a strong religious faith (34 per cent compared with 19 per cent) and more women than men said they believed in some sort of life after death (60 per cent compared with 39 per cent) but there was no difference in their denomination.

Asked whether their religious faith had been a help to them over their bereavement 93 per cent of the relatives who said they had a strong faith said it had. This is similar to the comparable proportion for the people who had died. But 48 per cent of the relatives with only some faith felt it had been a help compared with fewer, 36 per cent, of the people who died. An analysis by whether or not they had a religious faith and its strength revealed no associations with their feelings after bereavement over missing the person who died, loneliness, being able to look forward to things in the same way as they used to and whether they felt they had come to terms with the death of the person who died yet. But more of those with either a strong or some religious faith felt that the way things were going for them around the time they were interviewed was reasonable: 87 per cent compared with 78 per cent.

Another question that varied with their religious faith was their assessment of the quality of their relationship with the person who died. This is shown in Table 4.6. Those with no religious faith were less likely to describe their relationship with the person who died as "very good", and the proportion describing the relationship as only "fairly good" or "poor" was 3 per cent among those with a strong religious faith, 11 per cent among those with some or none. The differences between the sexes in their religious faith could not account for these variations as men and women relatives assessed the nature of their relationship with the person who died in similar ways.

Belief in some sort of life after death also seemed to be associated with a better assessment of their relationship with the person who died: 80 per cent of those who had such a belief described the relationship as "very good", 69 per cent of those who had not. Forty seven per cent of the "believers" compared with 31 per cent of the "non believers" felt loneliness was currently a problem for them. But when it came to an assessment of whether or not they felt they had come to terms with the death of the person who died yet there was no difference between those who believed in some sort of life after death and those who did not: it was those who were uncertain about this who were least likely to feel they had come to terms with it: 56 per cent compared with 69 per cent of the other two groups.

Table 4.6
Variation in reported quality of relationship between relative and the person who died with the religious faith of the relative

	Relative's religious faith			
Relatives' assessments of their relationship with the person who died	Strong %	Some %	None %	All* %
Very good	81	78	62	77
Good	15	12	18	14
Fairly good	3	7	10	6
Poor	-	2	7	2
Other comment	1	1	3	1
Number of relatives (=100%)	148	285	77	521

*Includes some for whom the strength of their faith was not known.

Conclusion

Some religious faith seemed to be more common among the people who died and among their bereaved relatives than in the general population, if Davis and Jowell's (1989) figure of 34 per cent is compared with the much higher figures in the 1987 study. Part of the difference may be explained by the older age of both the people who died and their relatives. But it could be that both approaching death and experience of bereavement stimulate religious belief.

The question of whether or not religion is a help around the time of death cannot be answered with any certainty. Most of those with a strong religious belief were thought to have been helped by it but, of course, these reports are likely to be influenced by people's expectations and perceptions. People who have a religious belief themselves may expect and indeed want to see religious faith as being helpful. People perceived as accepting their death may as a consequence have been thought to have a strong religious faith that enabled them to do so. Belief in some sort of life after death may not give rise to the same sort of expectation. This is suggested by the apparent lack of association between belief in some sort of life after death and the acceptance of death. Over this it appeared that uncertainty was more troubling than either a positive or negative belief.

Data about the relatives' own beliefs are likely to be more reliable than their perceptions about the faith of the people who died. But even so those with a religious faith probably have some vested interest in perceiving it as helpful. The lack of relationship between the religious belief of the relatives and most of the indicators of adjustment to bereavement is possibly more revealing. Another study (Bowling and Cartwright 1982) reported a rather similar finding. The association between relatives' assessments of the quality of their relationship with the person who died and their religious faith can be perceived as indicating that religious belief fosters good relationships or makes people more tolerant or more hypocritical.

Notes

1. Neighbours, friends who did not regard themselves as close to the deceased, staff of residential homes coroners and other officials were not asked these questions, so these data relate to 541 deaths.

5 The experience of caring

Changes in the household composition of the elderly in Britain were described in chapter one. Dale et al. (1987) explain the trend towards living alone, or with a spouse only, as being caused largely by increases in life expectancy, but also suggest that a fall in the age at marriage between 1945 and 1968, meaning that young people left home at earlier ages left more of the elderly living without their children. The consequences of these changes for the sources of support for those in need of care has been a cause for concern in a number of recent studies (Arber et al. 1988, Lewis and Meredith 1988, Qureshi and Walker 1989). These have also focused on how gender is related to the need for care, and to who performs the tasks of caring. As noted in chapter one, elderly widows living on their own form an increasingly high proportion of the elderly population although Timaeus (1986) suggests that this may not increase a great deal in the near future. The observation that the majority of care is provided by women has become commonplace (Allan 1988, Lewis and Meredith 1988, Qureshi and Walker 1989), and is only partially offset by Arber and Gilbert's (1988) analysis of General Household Survey data that shows the substantial amount of caring done by men in some situations.

Most people who die in Britain are elderly (79 per cent in 1986 were 65 and over and 55 per cent 75 and over [OPCS 1989b]) so studies of those who die are necessarily studies that focus largely on the needs of the elderly. However, the literature on care of the dying is disproportionately biased towards those with a recognisably terminal illness - almost always cancer - and those who die of cancer are, on average, significantly younger than those dying of other conditions (Seale 1989), containing a larger proportion of the "young elderly" rather than those over 75. Nevertheless, studies of the care of the terminally ill at home show the changes in household composition evident in the wider population: in 1952 the Joint National Cancer Survey

Committee found 7 per cent of people with terminal cancer living alone. Ward's study in 1985 found 22 per cent.

Here we describe the stresses of caring, which can be evaluated in the light of the concern of some authors (Lewis and Meredith 1988, Qureshi and Walker 1989) that government policy has led to an increase of pressure on carers. Concerns about the event of death itself - particularly the problem of dying alone in hospital - are explored, and the need for and receipt of care for those who are bereaved, who are often themselves elderly and now living alone, are described.

Households and family composition

Table 1.4 showed an increase in the proportion of respondents who were officials of residential homes, from 3 per cent in 1969 to 10 per cent in 1987. This reflects the increased proportion of people living and dying in institutional care. However, most respondents in 1987 were relatives, 36 per cent being spouses and 29 per cent being children or childrens' spouses. Ten per cent were friends or neighbours. While much of this chapter reports information given by all respondents, where relevant, certain categories of respondents, or of the deceased, are excluded from the analysis.

As was shown earlier (Table 2.2) the proportion living alone had more than doubled, rising from 15 per cent in 1969 to 32 per cent, and those living with a spouse only had also gone up, though not significantly, from 32 per cent to 38 per cent. Those living with others had declined in numbers, from 53 per cent to 30 per cent. These trends are similar to those in the population of over 65 year olds as a whole, described by Dale et al. (1987). The trend towards living alone was largely due to the greater numbers of women living alone. In the 1969 study only 19 per cent of women in the sample lived alone and 10 per cent of men. In 1987, 44 per cent of the women lived alone and 20 per cent of men. For men, an increased number lived with their spouse only (50 per cent in 1987 compared with 37 per cent in 1969). Women were less likely to live in families with their spouse and other people (15 per cent in 1969; 8 per cent in 1987). Concern about elderly widows living on their own would seem to be highly relevant for the population in their last year of life.

Table 5.1 demonstrates that people living alone in the 1987 sample were in a particularly unfortunate situation for potential sources of help. These people were least likely to have any children or siblings and were most likely to be widowed or divorced and old. The restrictions they suffered from (discussed in more detail later) were not at the highest level of any group, but over a fifth of them (the highest proportion of all groups) spent

Table 5.1
Household composition by family composition, restrictions, age, sex, marital status, cause of death and where lived (1987)[*]

	Alone %	With spouse only %	With spouse & others %	With others only %	All %
No children alive	42	19	0	34	26
No siblings alive	49	26	23	27	33
Restriction reported	57	61	54	65	59
Restriction for more than one year	33	31	18	38	31
Age 75+	68	43	18	58	50
Female	68	32	27	69	49
Married	1	99	99	2	52
Widowed/Divorced	83	1[a]	1[b]	64	37
Single	16	0	0	34	11
Died of cancer	19	39	42	27	31
Spent some time in old peoples' or nursing home	21	7	3	12	12
Total	163	191	71	83	508

[*]Excludes sudden deaths of people aged under 65 and people living in institution all year.

[a]Two spouses died in the year

[b]One person separated during the year.

some time in an old people's or nursing home. The results in Table 5.3, presented later, suggest that people living alone are the group most likely to progress to institutional care, as staff of residential homes or other officials were most often reported as bearing the brunt of caring for this group.

An example of a person who progressed to institutional care was that of an 84 year old widow who was mentally confused and lived on her own, being visited every day by her two daughters, one of whom always spent the day with her. Her daughter said:

> She was very confused, she really did not know day from night... she used to burn the kettles out (when she tried to make herself a hot drink) and used to hold (the telephone) the wrong way up... If we had night help we wouldn't have let her go in the home but she was so afraid at night that she said she wanted to go into a home... we used to visit every day and do things for her as if she was in her own home.

She was in the home less than three months when she fell and broke her leg, dying later in hospital of a pulmonary embolism.

Those living with others, but without a spouse, were the next oldest group, although this type of household was about half as common as those living alone. They were also quite likely to be elderly widows and to be single people but, perhaps because they were somewhat more likely than those living alone to have children or siblings alive, they could live with them when they started becoming restricted. In fact this group reported the highest proportion of long term restriction, a condition which, if they were living alone, would have meant a larger proportion entering institutional care.

Those living with their spouse only were the next most elderly group, as well as this being the most common type of household. With an average level of restriction, and being more likely than average to have children alive, their prospects both in terms of need for help and for sources on which they could draw, were better than the previous two groups. These people were more likely to be men, and this was even more likely to be true with the youngest group; those living with their spouse and others. This last group was the smallest, but all had children alive and less than a fifth experienced long term restriction.

Clearly, this pattern of household composition and gender is produced largely because women outlive their husbands more frequently than the reverse. Death from cancer, a disease with relatively short term but intense symptoms and restrictions when compared to the average of all other causes of death, also contributes to the pattern as it is a disease which strikes a younger age group than average (see chapter nine). It seems perverse to suggest that people dying from cancer - the focus of the hospice movement

Table 5.2
Restrictions reported for people who spent some part of their last year at home (sudden deaths under 65 excluded)

Could s/he manage to do these things without help?	Proportion needing help	% of those needing help who needed it for > a year	N
	%	%	(=100%)
Get in and out of bath or shower	52	48	(259)
Dress and undress	34	36	(174)
Go to toilet	30	26	(149)
Wash (and shave)	29	28	(148)
Feed self	17	26	(85)
Cut own toenails	57	64	(268)
Make self a hot drink	35	39	(172)
Did s/he need help at night	35	35	(166)
Any other things needed help with	24	53	(111)
Needed help with one or more of above (toenails excluded)	65	52	(297)
Total number of deaths	519		

and much of the research literature on the care of the dying - are lucky, but in terms of the help they can expect to receive from family members during their last year of life they are relatively fortunate.

Needs

In chapter two (Table 2.5) changes in the symptoms from which people in two samples suffered were reported. The incidence of symptoms in general did not show an increase or a decrease between 1969 and 1987, with some being more common (pain, constipation) and some less common (sleeplessness and loss of bowel control). However, the duration of time over which mental confusion, depression and incontinence were experienced had risen. These increases were all related to the greater proportion of people aged 75 or more in the 1987 study.

Unfortunately, comparison between the two studies for the level of restrictions cannot be made, as different questions were asked. However, the data for 1987 are presented in Table 5.2. The most common problem was with cutting toenails, and this was also the one most likely to be experienced on a long term basis. Getting into the bath or shower was the second most common and was also highly likely to be experienced on a long term basis. Nearly two thirds of the sample had some form of restriction, and over half of these had a problem (excluding toenails) for more than a year.

While it is likely that the need for care in the last year of life has risen since 1969, it is important to note that a large proportion (35 per cent) suffered no significant restriction while at home, and this is true of those 65 and over (32 per cent) and, to a lesser extent, of those 75 and over (27 per cent).

Who helped at home

Where respondents reported the presence of one or more of the restrictions listed in Table 5.2 they were asked who helped with these, and who had borne the brunt of care. The answers about who bore the brunt of care for the 298 people who experienced restriction at home are presented in Table 5.3.

Daughters caring for their elderly parents have been the focus of attention for a number of researchers working on the general topic of the care of the elderly (Allan 1988, Lewis and Meredith 1988, Qureshi and Walker 1989). In relation to this sample, however, this situation was most common for those living alone or in households without a spouse, both of these being households where the person who died was more likely to be an elderly widow. Otherwise, spouses played a larger part in care. In fact, spouses, overall, were more likely than children to bear the brunt of care and this is consistent with the findings of other studies involving samples of people who have died. The 1952 Joint National Cancer Survey Committee found that 40 per cent of the main carers in a sample of terminal cancer cases being looked after at home, were spouses. In the 1969 study of *Life before Death* the same figure was found for a random sample of adult deaths, and a similar local sample drawn by Wilkes (1984) found 50 per cent. Ward's (1985) study of cancer sufferers at home found 54 per cent and West et al (1986) found 71 per cent in their study of people with cancer. However, although daughters did not feature in caring to the extent suggested by studies of the elderly, the bias towards women taking on most of the care is evident in the figures in Table 5.3, and this is consistent with studies of elderly populations (Allan 1988, Arber et al. 1988, Lewis and Meredith 1988, Qureshi and Walker 1989).

Household composition was related in other ways to the main source of care. The data in Table 5.3 show that those living alone were particularly dependent on officials - such as district nurses or home helps - as well as friends and neighbours for care at home. This was less true for those living with others only, who were most likely to receive care from relatives other than spouses or children.

The figures for the overall number of relatives and friends helping vary with household composition, with those living alone having the fewest, and those with spouse and others the most. The average number of relatives and friends helping in 1987 (2.0) was significantly lower than for 1969, when the figure was three. Clearly demographic change is largely responsible for this.

Table 5.3
Who bore the brunt of caring for those with restrictions, by household composition*

	Alone	With spouse only	With spouse & others	With others only	All
	%	%	%	%	%
Wife	0	56	53	0	28
Husband	1	29	31	2	16
Daughter	23	3	11	29	15
Son	6	1	0	16	5
Other relative	11	1	0	33	9
Friend or neighbour	20	1	0	5	7
Official	38	7	0	11	16
More than one person	2	2	5	4	3
Total number of deaths (=100%)	94	120	38	55	307
Average number of relatives and friends who helped	1.7	1.9	3.1	2.0	2.0

*Excludes sudden deaths under 65 and those in an institution for a year or more before death.

The effect on those who bore the brunt of care[1]

Qureshi and Walker (1989) have presented powerful arguments against policies that force people to provide care to their dependent elderly relatives, describing the harmful effects that coercion can have on the caring relationship. The strain that such a pressure imposes is compounded where carers themselves have health problems. In the 1987 sample 45 per cent of relatives and friends who said they bore the brunt of care reported health problems which had made it difficult to do things for the person they were looking after. The physical strain of nursing the person who died would often then become extreme. One woman whose husband had died of lung cancer after a stroke the previous year said:

> I have arthritis. Apart from that I was just exhausted... it was all getting too much for me; I was becoming more and more exhausted... I did it willingly because he needed the care and I was his wife, but as he got worse I was getting worse as well and when he started to get awkward and refuse to go into hospital I got past it all and just rang the doctor and said I could not cope. I felt as though I was going to die myself.

Forty two per cent of those bearing the brunt said that either they or the deceased could have done with more help with the restrictions the deceased had suffered from. Thus, a daughter who nursed her 71 year old father who died of a brain tumour said:

> No one helped when dad was very ill. I've found out since that I could have had help from the hospice... I didn't know about it. I could have had a lot more help if I'd known... the district nurse came *once* and said "Are you happy to do what you're doing?" I said, I suppose so, so no one came again. As far as I'm concerned, the social services and social workers are the biggest con.

The friend of a woman dying of cancer said:

> She really needed someone there all the time to help her because she became very weak but she was very independent. After... she collapsed, a social worker came to see her. She got her a home help for one hour a week. That was neither here nor there.

The friend of a man living on his own in sheltered housing said:

He did have a home help but that was a waste of time. She never really cleaned the flat. She used to go out shopping, which wasn't necessary. He needed more time, more than two hours a week and he could have done with a bath nurse and meals on wheels.

Shortfalls in support from the formal services were not the only ones that carers identified. Twenty seven per cent of all respondents who helped with care said that there were relatives who might have helped more or visited more often.

The social isolation of carers has been identified (Allan 1988) as an important factor both in tying the carer to the relationship, and in producing feelings of resentment and guilt. Looking after the people who died placed restrictions on the lives of relatives and friends who bore the brunt of care. Sixty six per cent gave up or did less visiting of friends or relatives, the same for going out on social activities; 56 per cent gave up or did less going on holiday and 53 per cent entertaining at home. Twenty six per cent reported giving up or doing less work, and if people aged 65 or over are excluded from the total, as they might be presumed to be not in work anyway, the figure rises to 36 per cent. Over a third (36 per cent) said that their lives had been severely restricted, and only 16 per cent said they had suffered no restriction as a result of looking after the person who died.

Nevertheless, when asked whether looking after the deceased had been rewarding, a burden or equally balanced, 46 per cent of respondents who were relatives or friends who bore the brunt said they found it rewarding, and only seven per cent described it as a burden, 26 per cent saying it was a balance and the rest making some other comment. One daughter, who had looked after her mother for 11 years and described it as rewarding, said at this point:

> She did such a lot for me when I was young... she brought me up herself... I had double pneumonia when six years old and TB in the knee joints when I was little and didn't go to school for three years... My mother pushed me once a month up to the hospital in a long bath chair... She was wonderful to me. I'm just paying her back for all she did for me. She was working to earn a living as well, made dresses... she had a very hard life but I loved her very much.

Mixed feelings about caring have been described by Lewis and Meredith (1989), who refer to "a mixture of labour and love" and "the mixed legacy of satisfaction overlaid with bitterness." Allan (1988) has suggested that feelings of resentment can lead to the perception that "freedom will only come through the death of the old person."

In the present sample, of course, the dependent person had died, so it was possible to ask respondents whether they felt the person had died at the best time, or whether it would have been better if they had died earlier or later. Sixty one per cent of relatives and friends who bore the brunt of care felt the person had died at the right time, 22 per cent that earlier would have been better, and 11 per cent later, six per cent making some other comment. People who felt that looking after the person who died was a burden were no more likely than others to say that an earlier death would have been better. In fact, this sentiment was associated with indicators of poor quality of life in the person who died, which suggests that respondents either had only altruistic feelings, or suppressed any resentment about caring for the purposes of the interview. Where the quality of life of the person who died was judged to have been poor during their last year, 46 per cent of relatives and friends who bore the brunt of care felt that an earlier death would have been better, as opposed to nine per cent of those who felt the person's quality of life was good or fair.

One man, who died of cancer, was severely restricted in what he could do for himself for over three months before he died and suffered from a number of symptoms, including "very distressing" levels of pain. His widow felt his quality of life was poor and that an earlier death would have been better: "That last few months he was not well and had a lot of pain. He was just hanging on, but it was not the husband I had had the rest of the time." Another respondent who felt the same way was the niece of a man who had been "crippled with arthritis for years." She said: "If you are talking about quality of life, well the last year was not good at all. He was just existing, and in pain, so from that point of view I feel better earlier, but I don't know what he felt. I never heard him say he wanted to die." Another said of her husband who had died of mouth cancer: "He couldn't eat, he couldn't talk, he was in such pain. He suffered so much: it was awful, really awful."

Being there at the time of death

Bowling (1983) has presented a critique of the "hospitalisation of death" focusing in particular on the event of death itself, and arguing that the trend towards dying in hospital rather than home means that too many people die alone. However, dying alone, in the present sample, was actually less common for those dying in hospital (where 22 per cent died alone) than at home, where 31 per cent died alone. People who died from cancer were more likely to die alone if they were in hospital (24 per cent compared with 7 per cent of people dying with cancer at home), but this was true of no other major cause of death, the differences being in the opposite direction:

21 per cent of those not dying of cancer in hospital died alone, as opposed to 42 per cent of such people dying at home. People dying of stroke, ischaemic heart disease and other circulatory conditions showed the largest difference between home and hospital. These conditions are more likely to cause sudden death, and in the case of stroke, to be associated with living alone. The distress for people dying alone can only be guessed at; relatives too may be deprived of the opportunity to say goodbye, with harmful consequences for their subsequent coping with bereavement. Only just over a third (37 per cent) of the respondents who were relatives and friends were with the person when they died. Of those who were not there, 61 per cent would have liked to have been. One man said of the time his wife died in hospital of heart failure while he was not present: "That's what hurts the most. I was playing golf. I didn't want to believe that she was so bad."
Another respondent, the wife of a man who collapsed in the home having had a heart attack said: "I always wonder, if I'd been there, could I have done anything? Even ring for an ambulance."

In fact, 24 per cent of the people who died did so alone. People who lived alone were the most likely to die alone: 36 per cent did so, as opposed to 20 per cent of others living in private households. Some were only found when the smell from their rooms became noticeable. A man who lived alone committed suicide with an overdose of paracetamol. His neighbour said:

> I used to go into my back bedroom and there was an awful smell in there. I reported it to housing... the smell got worse so I reported it again. Then I came home one afternoon and my wife said the police had been... and broken in. They found his body, badly decomposed... They reckon he had been dead for five or six weeks.

In two other instances similar to this, the only person that could be found to give an interview for the survey was an environmental health officer.

In spite of the increasing frequency of death in hospital, there was no evidence to suggest that respondents felt that it would have been better for the death to have occurred elsewhere. Where the person died at home, respondents were asked whether they felt it would have been better if the person had been in a hospital or other institution. Twelve per cent of those who were relatives and friends said they felt this way. But the same proportion of respondents for people dying in hospitals or hospices felt that it would have been better to have the person at home at the time of death. On the whole, the decision to admit to hospital, perhaps because of growing difficulties in coping at home, were felt to be justified.

Bereavement and adjustment to loss[2]

Losing the person who died meant that many of the respondents were themselves now living alone. Of 311 relatives and friends who were respondents who used to live with the deceased, 63 per cent had now to adjust to living alone. Spouses were particularly likely to be in this position; 70 per cent of respondents who were spouses were living alone at the time of interview compared with 22 per cent of other types of respondent. Although widows were not significantly more likely to be living alone than widowers, they were more numerous (68 per cent of respondents widowed by the death were female).

Respondents reported themselves experiencing a number of symptoms that had been caused or made worse by the deceased's illness and death. Forty one per cent reported sleeplessness, 44 per cent nerves or depression and 20 per cent loss of appetite. Spouses were more likely to suffer from these things than other respondents (24 per cent reported all three of these, as opposed to 6 per cent of other relatives and friends) and widows more than widowers (28 per cent compared to 15 per cent). Sixty two per cent of respondents had consulted a doctor since the person had died and of these 37 per cent were prescribed something to help them sleep or feel less miserable.

Table 5.4 presents data that indicate respondents' adjustment to bereavement, according to their relationship to the deceased. Once again, the situation of spouses stands out as one of particular difficulty, as on all the

Table 5.4
Adjustment to death

	Spouses	Other relatives /friends*
	%	%
Miss a great deal	84	56
Not come to terms with death	39	15
Loneliness is a big problem	26	7
Cannot look forward to things in the same way	70	23
Things altogether going not very well/ not well at all	16	11
Total number of deaths	231	308

*Excludes friends who were not close

indicators of adjustment in Table 5.4 spouses were more likely to be doing badly. There were no significant differences for these indicators between widows and widowers.

One widower who felt that things were not going at all well said: "I get up in the mornings and I don't feel like doing anything. You come down on your own and the day is so long. You sweep up or go shopping and I think "why did she go?" I start thinking about her and upset myself. A widow said: "There's no one here at all; even the cat's gone off... I've got a different life... I don't know what to do... things aren't the same... (I get lonely) at night time. It gets me down all by myself."

Support for the bereaved[2]

Eighty four per cent of respondents claimed some religious faith, and 64 per cent said they had found it helpful in coping with their bereavement. In fact, ministers of religion were the most frequent visitors to the bereaved of any professional group (37 per cent of respondents were visited), almost twice as many as were visited by their own general practitioner (19 per cent). Nurses visited 10 per cent and social workers 6 per cent. However, this may reflect the greater willingness of ministers of religion to visit the home compared to general practitioners, because when asked with whom they had talked about their feelings about the death, 29 per cent of respondents mentioned their general practitioner, more than had been visited at home by one. The figure for ministers of religion was 23 per cent, suggesting that their visits did not always result in the exploration of emotions. In fact, the people that most respondents said they had talked to were not professionals, but their own relatives (77 per cent) or friends (55 per cent).

Fifteen per cent of respondents had talked to no one about their feelings, but this did not seem to be a problem for them as these people were no more likely than others to say that they would have liked to talk to someone (or someone else). Overall, 10 per cent of respondents still felt they wanted someone to talk to.

One such person was a woman of 47 whose husband had died of a heart attack. She had been visited by various professionals, and had talked with them as well as friends and relations about her feelings but she still felt a need to talk that was not being met:

> (Some) neighbours and friends... think after a few months I should be OK... I found when I went back to work people think "Oh, she's alright now," and I'm not. It's really only the beginning... I need to talk. It's a funny thing: I had lots of friends but I haven't now. Some won't talk

about it, and neighbours too. I think they don't know what to say. I can understand in a way. At first they didn't know what to say but even now if they just said, "How are you? How are you feeling?" But some neighbours cross the road if they see me. I can't understand it.

Conclusion

Demographic changes since 1969 have meant that both for those in their last year of life and for those caring for people who die, fewer family resources are available. The household and family composition of the elderly, who form the majority of the population in their last year of life, have changed so that more people live alone now, or with their spouse only, and have less access to care from relatives than was previously the case. Elderly widows are particularly disadvantaged in this respect, and the results illustrate the progression of events that so many of these widows will have experienced; from caring for a dependent husband, to bereavement and the difficulties of adjustment to living alone with grief and, perhaps, increasing dependency in themselves.

It has been argued (Johnson 1989) that the dependency of the elderly on their relatives has been overemphasized, at least in economic terms, and it may be that a view of the elderly as providers of care as well as receivers would help redress negative images of old age. Certainly, even in their last year of life a substantial proportion of the sample - and of the elderly within it - were not highly dependent on others for help. Those dying of cancer, who are the focus of much of the medical and nursing effort in providing new approaches to the care of the dying (Saunders and Baines 1983), are more fortunate than others in this respect. Their illness tends to be shorter term, if more intensely distressing, and those dying of cancer tend, because of their age, to be those with relatives available to help, and to be there at the time of death.

Nevertheless, the indicators of need in the present study suggest high levels of dependency in those in their last year of life, and such comparisons with 1969 that are possible suggest that dependency is experienced over a longer time period than before. The mixed feelings of carers, from guilt and resentment through to feelings of obligation and love, are amply demonstrated, although the balance seems to be in favour of altruism, as the desire for dependants to die sooner is uncommon.

Above all, the results demonstrate the disadvantage that women suffer at this stage of life, both as dependants and carers. More of the people who are most dependent live alone, with few sources of informal care, and these tend to be women. Women are most likely to take on the main burden of caring, particularly where they are spouses, who are often themselves elderly with health problems. These same women are amongst those most likely to be living alone after the death, and although the grief of bereaved spouses is equal for both sexes, the greater number of women surviving their husbands ensure that once again women are disproportionately likely to suffer.

Finally, this chapter demonstrates the value of a perspective on death and dying that is not narrowly confined to cancer, hitherto the focus of much of the medical and nursing innovations of the hospice movement (Saunders and Baines 1983). Most people do not die of cancer (OPCS 1989b). The problems of the dying share much with the problems of the elderly population.

Notes

1. Relatives and friends who said they bore the brunt of care are considered in this section; others are excluded except where indicated otherwise.

2. This section concerns relatives and friends only, except where indicated otherwise.

6 Social class differences

Social class differences in mortality persist (DHSS Working Group 1980, Blane et al. 1990, Davey-Smith et al. 1990) and it appears that most of the differentials must be attributed to socioeconomic environment, lifestyles and circumstances before death rather than to changing social class as a result of ill health (Fox et al. 1985). If poverty and deprivation are the main causes of premature death and lesser life expectancy in the lower social classes (Morris 1990), what impact do these have on the quality and circumstances of life before death? To what extent do people in different social classes have different health problems, receive different sorts of care and experience different types of deprivation in the year before they die?

The 1969 study found no social class differences in reported symptoms or restrictions or the type of help people needed except that working class people more often needed financial help. There were also clear variations in housing conditions and household equipment with social class. In this chapter we examine the nature and extent of class differences in a range of circumstances at this stage of life, and see whether the same pattern of similarity and variation still persists.[1]

Class differences

National statistics show clear social class trends in the standardized mortality rates and in the years of potential life lost (Blane et al. 1990). Table 6.1 shows that in the 1987 sample of deaths a higher proportion of the middle class ones occurred at ages 75 or more: 60 per cent compared with 50 per cent of working class deaths; and more working class deaths occurred under 65: 25 per cent compared with 17 per cent.

Table 6.1
Social class differences in health, care and circumstances in the year before death

	Middle class	Working class
Age at death		
Under 65	17%	25%
65 - 74	23%	25%
75 or more	60%	50%
	(192)*	(396)
Siblings alive at time of death	57%(183)	69%(376)
Died in residential home	17%(192)	10%(396)
Spent some of last year:		
in any residential home	27%(191)	19%(396)
in private residential home	15%(192)	9%(395)
in private hospital or hospice	7%(170)	1%(370)
Visited at home by general practitioner in last year	85%(162)	77%(349)
General practitioner felt to have time to discuss things	88%(148)	79%(285)
Had general practitioner who qualified in Great Britain	83%(149)	74%(307)

Table 6.1 continued

Needed help with feeding themselves for a year or more	2%(183)	6%(374)
Lived in a bungalow	17%(186)	10%(388)
Had telephone	95%(146)	79%(323)
Cost a problem in keeping home warm	7%(142)	15%(311)
Had received:		
supplementary benefit	12%(139)	26%(283)
heating allowance	4%(137)	13%(291)
rent or rate rebate	30%(142)	50%(293)
Thought to have needed more financial help	16%(136)	32%(292)
Described as having had a good quality of life in year before death	43%(165)	30%(335)

*The figures in brackets are the numbers on which the percentages are based (= 100%).

Certain exclusions have been made in some instances (see text).

The sample was too small to show class differences in cause of death but for cancer there was a difference in the expected direction that did not reach statistical significance: 23 per cent of the middle class deaths compared with 30 per cent of the working class ones were attributed to cancer.

Family and social circumstances Given their older age at death it might be thought that fewer of the middle class people would have a husband or wife who survived them although most of their spouses too would have a longer life expectancy. In practice there were no significant class differences in marital status but the proportions who were married at the time of their death were 43 per cent of the middle class, 49 per cent of the working class (a difference which did not reach statistical significance). More of the working class had brothers or sisters who were alive (69 per cent compared with 57 per cent) but there was no difference between the two groups in the proportion with living children (71 per cent overall) and the proportion living alone during the last year of their lives was similar (32 per cent altogether).[2]

Place of death A comparatively high proportion of middle class deaths took place in old people's homes or nursing homes: 17 per cent compared with 10 per cent of working class deaths. The difference between the two groups remained if the comparison is restricted to deaths of people aged 85 or more for which the proportions were 47 per cent and 25 per cent. In relation to this, staff of residential homes were more often interviewed about the deaths of middle class than those of working class people: 13 per cent compared with 6 per cent. There were no other class differences in place of death.

Admission to residential homes Similar proportions of middle and working class people who died, 8 per cent, had spent at least some of the last year of their lives in residential homes that were run by local authorities, but more middle class people had spent some of this time in private residential homes (15 per cent compared with 9 per cent) and the proportions spending time in any residential home (including those run by charities and other organizations) was 27 per cent of the middle class, and 19 per cent of the working class. None of the questions asked about amenities and conditions in the residential homes revealed any significant class difference although 70 per cent of middle class residents compared with 53 per cent of working class ones had had a room of their own, a difference which did not quite reach statistical significance.

Home nursing care People in residential homes received similar amounts of care from domiciliary nurses as others (see chapter eleven) but as in the earlier, 1969 study older people and those dying from cancer were more likely to have received help at home from a nurse (see chapter fifteen). As the middle class people who died were older, but rather more of the working class people died of cancer it might be expected that these tendencies would cancel each other out, and so it appeared to be: the same proportion of middle and working class people, 42 per cent, had had some help from a nurse at home in the 12 months before they died. Among those who had not had any help similar proportions of both social class groups (11 per cent overall) were thought to have needed it. Among those receiving help rather more of the working than of the middle class had had this help for six months or more, 43 per cent compared with 29 per cent, but there was no significant difference in the frequency with which the help was given, or in the type of care received. When asked to describe the help and care the dying people got from nurses as excellent, good, fair or poor rather more of the respondents for working class people opted for fair or poor: 16 per cent compared with 6 per cent of respondents for middle class people.

Hospitals and hospices Similar proportions of both middle and working class people had been admitted to a hospital or hospice during the last year of their lives and they had spent similar lengths of time there, but more of the middle class had been in private hospitals or hospices: seven per cent compared with one per cent. In addition more of the middle class people had had a room of their own at some stage of their stay in hospital (41 per cent compared with 29 per cent), but if this analysis is confined to stays in NHS hospitals or hospices only the difference is no longer significant (36 per cent compared with 28 per cent). There were no differences between the two groups in the respondents' assessments of the care they had received in hospital. Neither was there any difference in the proportion who had had a domiciliary consultation (a home visit from a doctor based in a hospital or hospice), which was 14 per cent overall.

Contact with general practitioners The observation that rather more of the middle class than of the working class people who died had been visited at home by a general practitioner in the last year of their lives (85 per cent compared with 77 per cent) can be attributed to the older age of the middle class people; when age was controlled for there was no significant difference. Assessments of the care given by general practitioners were also similar for the two groups except that respondents for middle class people were more likely to feel that the general practitioner had had time to discuss things: 88 per cent compared with 79 per cent. Other studies have found that general practitioner consultation times were rather longer with middle class than with working class patients (Buchan and Richardson 1973, Cartwright and O'Brien 1976).

Analyses by various characteristics of the doctors - age, sex, membership of the Royal College of General Practitioners, whether or not the doctor was a registered trainer, average size of list, and country of qualification - revealed one class difference: the middle class people who died were more likely to have had a doctor who qualified in Great Britain: 83 per cent compared with 74 per cent of the working class people who died. A similar class difference was observed on a study of general practice (Cartwright and Anderson 1981) covering a wider sample.

Symptoms and restrictions It might be expected that because of their greater age at death middle class people would suffer from more of the symptoms that increase with age. Symptoms which have been shown to do this among those aged 65 or more are constipation, confusion, drowsiness or dry mouth, incontinence, difficulty seeing and hearing (Cartwright 1990). None of these, or any of the other 16 specific symptoms asked about, were reported significantly more often for middle class than for working class people. But one of them, a dry mouth, was reported for 37 per cent of working class people, but only 28 per cent of middle class ones. It is a symptom which is often a side effect of medicine taking but there is no evidence that working class people take more medicines than middle class people (Cartwright and Smith 1988). A significant difference in one out of 16 symptoms might have occurred just by chance. In addition to not having more symptoms than working class people, there was no indication that middle class people had had the symptoms that were reported for longer.

Our enquiries into restrictions were concerned with the person's ability to do the things listed below without help in the period before death or before going into a hospital or hospice for the last time.

> Get in and out of a bath or shower
> Dress and undress including shoes and fastenings
> Go to the toilet and cope on own when there
> Wash (and shave)
> Feed him or herself
> Cut own toenails
> Make him or herself a hot drink
> Help needed at night
> Help needed with any other thing

More of the working class people who died were reported to have needed help with feeding themselves for a year or more: 6 per cent compared with two per cent of middle class people. There were no other class differences.

Housing[3] More middle class than working class people who died had had a telephone: 95 per cent compared with 79 per cent, but similar proportions (72 per cent overall) had a washing machine. For almost a quarter (23 per cent) of both groups their home was described as not an easy place for them, and no significant differences emerged when respondents were asked whether there were any problems with the position of the lavatory (18 per cent), the distance from the shops (16 per cent) or the stairs (35 per cent reported difficulties) although more middle class people had lived in bungalows: 17 per cent compared with 10 per cent. But more of the working than of the middle class were said to have had some other housing problem (12 per cent compared with 5 per cent). Illustrations of the difficulties reported were:

> Not enough room after the bed had been brought downstairs. There was only one living room and with the bed in it it didn't leave much room for others (wife and son). We had to bring it downstairs because he couldn't walk upstairs and the toilet was downstairs anyway and there was no heating upstairs. (Son of man who died of lung cancer).

> Her flat was on the top, third floor. It was too high up. She couldn't manage the stairs. She just never went out. The council could have helped by moving her into sheltered housing on the ground floor. That's what she really needed, to be in a flat where there was a warden to look after her. I tried to get her in but was told there was nowhere for her. (Sister of woman who lived alone and died of heart failure aged 65-74).

Some of the problems could have been overcome by money and 15 per cent of the working class compared with 7 per cent of the middle class reckoned that cost was a problem in keeping the person's home warm enough.

Finance Apart from any difficulties over heating their homes 11 per cent of the working class compared with 6 per cent of the middle class were said to have had other financial problems. There was no difference between the two groups in the proportions who had had a mobility allowance (8 per cent had one), an attendance allowance (15 per cent) a disability pension (6 per cent), or financial help from relatives (10 per cent), but more of the working class had had supplementary benefit (26 per cent compared with 12 per cent), a heating allowance (13 per cent compared with 4 per cent) and a rent or rate rebate (50 per cent compared with 30 per cent). But in spite of these additional sources of help respondents felt that twice as many of the working class than of the middle class people who died could have done with more financial help: 32 per cent compared with 16 per cent. Clearly allowances are too low to overcome the financial problems faced by a substantial proportion of people in the months before their death: 40 per cent of those receiving supplementary benefit, 34 per cent of those with a rent or rate rebate and 44 per cent of those with a heating allowance were thought to have needed more financial help.

Communication[4] There were no differences between the middle and working class in the proportion thought to have known they were dying or to have known their diagnosis. Neither were there any differences in respondents' assessments about whether knowing or not knowing had been best as it was, or whether they themselves had been able to find out all they wanted to know, or in their main sources of information and support. Similar proportions of the two groups said they had talked to the person who died about his or her death (37 per cent had done so if the person was thought to have realised they were dying).

Quality of life and time of death Towards the end of the interview two questions were asked about the timeliness of death and the quality of the person's life in the year before death. In assessing the timeliness of death respondents were asked to take the person's illness into account and then say whether they thought the person had died at the best time or whether it would have been better if he or she had died earlier or later. Most, 59 per cent, people were thought to have died at the best time, for 22 per cent it was thought better if they had died earlier, for 13 per cent later and for 6 per cent there were other comments. There were no social class differences over this. Altogether 34 per cent of the people who died were described as having had a good quality of life in the year before their death; this proportion was higher for middle class than for working class people: 43 per cent compared with 30 per cent. The difference remained when deaths for which staff of residential homes were interviewed were excluded.

Conclusion

Given that middle class people had lived, on average, rather longer than working class people it might have been expected that middle class people would have more symptoms, be more restricted and have a generally poorer quality of life during the year before their death. None of these happened; on the contrary, middle class people were reported to have a rather better quality of life during this time. A contributory cause to this difference seemed to be money. More working class people were felt to be in financial need, and among those who were thought to need more financial help only 26 per cent were thought to have had a good quality of life compared with 38 per cent of those not in need. Other differences between middle and working class people that may have played a part were housing and possibly rather poorer care. Private hospitals and private residential homes were less accessible to working class people and this may be why they needed longer nursing care at home and also why more of them needed long term help with feeding before they died or went into hospital for the last time. Other indications that working class people may have received less good care were the higher level of criticism of the way they were looked after by domiciliary nurses, the apparent willingness of general practitioners to spend more time discussing things with middle class patients and the fact that middle class people were more likely to have general practitioners who trained in Great Britain.

In many ways the experiences of middle and working class people in the last year of their lives were remarkably similar: for the most part they suffered from the same symptoms and had the same restrictions, they spent similar lengths of time in hospitals where they were apparently cared for in similar ways. If their different ages are taken into account they were visited or neglected by their general practitioners to the same extent and they had similar communications problems, or lack of them.

The similarity of symptoms and restrictions although middle class people die at a later age suggest that working class people may be ageing earlier and be more subject to what Martin (1990) has described as the negative features of old age which can be traced to poverty and powerlessness. Some of the things that money can buy may postpone the ageing process and make the last year of life rather less unpleasant. The similarity of the findings in 1969 and 1987 support results from other studies about the persistence of social inequalities, but indicate that in the year before death these are more related to social circumstances than to health.

Notes

1. Data about occupation, or for married and widowed women their husband's occupation, were taken from the death registration forms and then classified by social class using the Classification of Occupations (OPCS 1980). Eight per cent of the deaths could not be classified in this way; three quarters of these were deaths of women. For analysis professional, intermediate and skilled non manual occupations have been taken as middle class and manual skilled, partly skilled and unskilled occupations as working class. Among those that could be classified 31

per cent of the male deaths were middle class, a similar proportion, 34 per cent of the female deaths. Classification of cause of death was also taken from the registration forms.

2. Those who had lived in an institution for a year or more before their death have been excluded from this last figure as the question was not asked about them.

3. Questions about housing and finance were not asked for people who died suddenly and without any restrictions before they were 65 or for those who had been in a hospital or other institutions for a year or more before they died.

4. Questions about communications and the quality of life and timeliness of death were not asked for people who died suddenly and with no restrictions before they were 65.

7 Old age

As was shown in chapter one, most deaths in this, as in other industrialised countries, occur to old people. Over a fifth of the deaths in England and Wales in 1990 were of people aged 85 or more, and four fifths were 65 or over (OPCS 1992a). Moreover, as a result of lower infant mortality rates, changes in life expectation and in the age distribution of the population, the average age at death is increasing. Between 1971 and 1991 the proportion of deaths to people aged 75 or more rose from just under 45 per cent to just over 58 per cent (OPCS 1992b).

But much of the discussion about care of the dying, and indeed much of the research in this field, focus on deaths from cancer. This is because such deaths are generally more predictable than those from other causes. In addition, hospice services cater largely for people with cancer. This emphasis on people dying from cancer means that the deaths of older people are relatively neglected in relation to both care and research. This is because those dying from cancer are comparatively young. In 1990 in England and Wales two out of five of the deaths of those aged 55-64 were attributed to cancer compared with one in eight of those aged 85 or more. Among all deaths this proportion was a quarter (OPCS 1992a).

In this chapter we try to redress the balance of much research by focusing on the deaths of older people and comparing the circumstances of the last year of their lives and the care they received with those of people dying at younger ages.

Table 7.1
Variations with age at death

Age at death	Under 55	55-64	65-74	75-84	85+
Respondent	%	%	%	%	%
Husband or wife	53	54	58	30	6
Son or daughter	10	15	18	32	39
Other relative	26	15	13	15	20
Friend or neighbour	6	7	9	12	12
Staff of home or other official	-	5	2	10	23
Other	5	4	-	1	-
Restriction in activities[a]					
No restrictions	57	54	40	32	8
Restrictions cutting toe nails only	-	1	4	8	6
Restrictions for:					
Less than 3 months	22	20	22	11	5
3 months < 1 year	9	13	8	13	8
1 year +	12	12	26	36	73
Where died					
Own home	32	41	34	16	14
Hospital	43	39	50	61	44
Hospice	5	5	5	4	-
Residential or nursing home	2	1	3	12	37
Other	18	14	8	7	5
General practitioner consultations in last year of life[a]					
Estimated average number of					
Home visits	5.3	4.9	5.9	6.9	9.5
Surgery consultations	4.4	4.5	3.5	3.0	1.1
Total consultations	9.7	9.4	9.4	9.9	10.6
Demographic & social circumstances					
Female	34%	39%	38%	56%	79%
Married	64%	65%	66%	39%	16%
With living siblings	92%	79%	77%	55%	41%
Some time in residential home	5%	3%	8%	24%	56%
All last year in residential home	2%	3%	1%	10%	37%
Living alone	9%	19%	24%	41%	50%
Total number of deaths[*]	62	80	147	203	147

[*]The proportion living alone excludes those living in an institution all year and sudden deaths of those under 65 with no restrictions.
[a]Those in hospital for a year or more before death excluded.

The effect of age

Family and living circumstances

Table 7.1 shows the respondents for people of different ages. For older people of 75 or more information was less likely to be obtained from husbands or wives, more often from sons or daughters but overall less often from any relatives and more frequently from the staff of residential homes. This is a reflection of changing demographic circumstances. As the table shows, older people who died were more often women and were less likely to be married and to have living siblings. In addition, older people of 85 or more were less likely to have any living children, 61 per cent compared with 74 per cent of people dying at younger ages. This may be because more of their children had died, it may also be a generational effect with the older cohort having smaller families and the women being less likely to marry as a result of the 1914-18 war. Twenty per cent of the women aged 85 or more had never married, compared with 12 per cent of the younger ones (though this difference was not statistically significant). So older people are less likely to have a spouse or a sibling or a son or daughter to care for them. They are much more likely to spend some or all of the last year of their lives in a residential home. But if they do not live in a residential home a much higher proportion live alone. These differences are also shown in Table 7.1.

Symptoms and restrictions

Turning to the symptoms they were reported to have experienced in the last year, the main finding is the lack of difference between people dying at different ages. Table 7.2 shows the symptoms with no significant age variation together with the proportion for which they were reported. It illustrates that dying at any age is generally preceded by a lot of unpleasant symptoms, an average of five of the symptoms in Table 7.2.

Table 7.3 shows the symptoms for which there were age variations. Mental confusion, incontinence, difficulty hearing and seeing and to a lesser, but still significant, extent, dizziness were all more common among people dying at later ages. Only a persistent cough was more often reported for people dying at younger ages. Taking all symptoms together, the number reported increased with age from 5.7 for those under 65 to 7.4 for those aged 85 or more. As might be expected, those dying at an older age had had their symptoms for longer: 69 per cent of the symptoms reported for those aged 85 or more were said to have lasted for a year or more compared with 39 per cent of those reported for people dying when they were under 65 and 52

Table 7.2
Symptoms for which no difference with age at death reported and proportion for whom symptom reported

Pain	72%	Dry mouth/thirst	33%
Trouble breathing	49%	Backache	31%
Loss of appetite	47%	Bad temper	23%
Drowsiness	44%	Difficulty swallowing	23%
Sleeplessness	40%	Bed sores	18%
Constipation	36%	Unpleasant smell	14%
Depression	36%	Dribbling	13%
Vomiting, feeling sick	33%		

Number of deaths (=100%) 639

Table 7.3
Symptoms with an age variation

Age at death	Under 55	55-64	65-74	75-84	85+
Mental confusion	21%	25%	26%	43%	52%
Loss of bladder control	24%	16%	24%	38%	51%
Loss of bowel control	19%	8%	19%	25%	32%
Difficulty seeing	10%	5%	19%	24%	46%
Difficulty hearing	4%	7%	20%	31%	54%
Dizziness	22%	18%	25%	38%	33%
Persistent cough	28%	30%	30%	17%	10%
Number of deaths (=100%)	62	80	147	203	147

per cent for the intermediate group aged 65-84. In contrast, those dying at an older age were less likely to be reported as finding their symptoms "very distressing." The proportion of symptoms described in this way fell from 50 per cent for those under 55 to 31 per cent for those aged 85 or more. This last difference might arise because of the different relationship between respondents and the people who died (staff of homes were generally found to take a relatively optimistic view of things [Cartwright and Seale 1990]), to different perceptions of distress among older and younger people, to a more stoical attitude among older people, to an adjustment to persistent and long lasting symptoms or to a real difference in the intensity of symptoms and the resulting level of distress.

People's ability to look after themselves showed a steep decline with age. (The activities asked about are indicated on p.82). Older people were not only more restricted in the things they could do before they died, they had also been restricted for longer (see Table 7.1).

With these restrictions it is not surprising that older people living at home and not in residential care, had more problems at home. The main differences, shown in Table 7.4, were between those under and over 85. Half of the latter had problems with the stairs and for a third the position of the lavatory presented some difficulty.

In addition the very old, aged 85 or more, were less likely to have a telephone at home; 71 per cent did so compared with 87 per cent of the people under that age, while the proportion with a washing machine was 53 per cent for those aged 85 or more, 64 per cent for those aged 75-84 and 84 per cent for those under 75.

Table 7.4
Problems with housing by age at death

	Under 85	85+
Home not an easy place	21%	35%
Difficulty with:		
Stairs	33%	49%
Position of lavatory	15%	33%
Distance from shops	14%	24%
Number of deaths(=100%)*	430	82

*Excludes those living in an institution all year, and sudden deaths of people under 65 with no restrictions about whom these questions were not asked.

Care

Home help services seemed responsive to the increasing needs of older people, and those living alone were much more likely to get help from this service than those living with others. The figures are in Table 7.5. However, in the respondents' views there was still a lot of unmet need for the home help service: among those living with others 35 per cent of those dying when they were 85 or more were thought to have needed some or more help compared with 16 per cent of those dying at a younger age, while among those living alone 34 per cent were thought to have some unmet need, but there was no significant variation in this proportion with age.

Older people of 75 or more were also more likely to make use of day centres in the final year of their lives than people dying at younger ages (see chapter twelve). In contrast, the estimated average number of all general practitioner consultations in the last 12 months of life hardly varied with age. Although home visits were higher among those aged 85 or more this was offset by the fall off in surgery consultations. This is shown in Table 7.1. People who lived alone had *fewer* consultations than those who lived with others (see chapter fourteen).

Nursing care at home, which was mainly provided by district nurses, showed no definite variation with age in the proportion receiving such care. The overall proportion was 41 per cent. But when respondents were asked whether the person could have done with any help from a nurse during the 12 months before they died more of those aged 85 or more who did not get any help were thought to have needed it: 22 per cent compared with 8 per cent for younger people.

In spite of their greater restrictions, and the increase with age of some symptoms, older people were not receiving more attention from general practitioners or from home nurses. As is shown in chapter ten people dying when they were 85 or more were the least likely to be admitted to a hospital or hospice in the last year of their lives; this in spite of the fact that more older people died from cerebro-vascular accidents, a cause of death associated with a high use of the hospital service.

Table 7.5
Proportion receiving care from home help services by age at death and whether living alone (excluding those in residential homes for year before death)

	Under 65	65-74	75-84	85+	All
Living alone	28%	26%	52%	73%	49%
	(18)	(34)	(67)	(41)	(160)
Living with others	8%	8%	15%	28%	12%
	(111)	(104)	(97)	(39)	(351)
All	11%	12%	30%	51%	24%
	(129)	(138)	(164)	(80)	(511)

Figures in brackets are the numbers on which the percentages are based (=100%)

Finally, people of 85 or more were less likely than those aged 65-84 to die in a hospital. None of the former died in a hospice and few in their own homes, over a third of them died in a residential or nursing home. This can be seen from Table 7.1.

Conclusion

The main finding in this chapter is that people dying when they are old have greater needs, less support from relatives and less medical and nursing care in relation to their needs than people dying at younger ages. Their needs are greater because they are less able to care for themselves, they also have rather more symptoms, particularly long term ones. The observation that their symptoms were rather less likely to be regarded by respondents as very distressing for the people who died may reflect a disturbing tolerance of distress for old people by those close to them or a genuine difference; a study based on information from the people themselves is needed to decide this.

The decline in the availability of wives, husbands, sisters and brothers and, for this particular cohort, daughters and sons, to care for them is accompanied by an increase in help from social services. But among those living alone, many of whom are elderly, and among those living with others and aged 85 or more there was still felt to be a substantial amount of unmet need for help with shopping, cooking and cleaning.

This results in many of the older people who die spending the last part of their lives in a residential home. Many of them will have been faced with a choice between an unpleasant battle to survive in their own homes and an unpleasant enforced dependence in an institution (Wilkin and Hughes 1987). Others will have had no choice (Allen 1992).

The most disconcerting finding from the study is the lack of responsiveness of the medical and nursing services to the needs of older people in the last year of their lives. There is some evidence that general practitioners, community nurses, hospitals and hospices all contribute to this. In chapter ten it is argued that there is a need for a critical review of the medical care of people in residential homes. An increasing number of studies are revealing the failure to give appropriate medical care to older people who would benefit from them (Berisa et al. 1989, Cook and Hubner 1989, Ormerod and Westaby 1988, Fentiman et al. 1990, Pell et al. 1990, Haig et al. 1991, Dixon 1992). This data in this chapter add to this mounting evidence.

Part II
HOSPICE, HOSPITAL AND INSTITUTIONAL CARE

Introduction

It will be clear by now that the availability of resources for informal care, in the form of family and friends willing and able to take on the task of looking after dependent people in the last year of life, has declined since 1969. In these circumstances, the role of formal services is increasingly important. In Part IV the issue of how to achieve the right balance between care for people in their own homes, and institutional care, will be discussed. In Part III, though, we consider peoples' experience of a variety of forms of institutional care.

As explained in the introductory chapter, the hospice movement has been an area of dramatic growth since the first study of *Life before Death*, and assessment of its influence on care of the dying in general was an important reason for doing the 1987 study. In one sense, this task is an impossible one since, as explained in the introductory chapter, the hospice movement itself is a reflection of broader changes in social and professional attitudes regarding death, which might be expected to have an independent influence on practice in hospitals, nursing homes and other places where those in the last year of life receive care.

However it is possible, given the study design, to place the contribution of the hospice movement in the context of death and dying in general. Firstly, the proportion of the dying who receive hospice services in Britain has not hitherto been possible to establish from official statistics. National records of place of death (for example, OPCS 1989b) do not distinguish hospices separately, and there are no national records of the extent of use of hospice services. Chapter eight, which is largely devoted to a comparison between people who died of cancer who received hospice services and those who did not, gives figures for this. Secondly, the chapter makes an assessment of the extent to which specialist hospice care is different from conventional hospital and domiciliary care of the terminally ill.

Although it is important to assess the direct effect of hospice care in this way, it will become clear that hospices in practice only serve a small minority of people who die. In chapter nine the contribution of the hospice movement is placed in a broader context, through a comparison of the characteristics of those who die from cancer, and those who die from other causes. Some of the themes that began to emerge in Part II are developed. These concern the effect of very old age on the experience of dying, and differences in communication issues when it is not possible to identify a clear moment at which a person becomes terminally ill. The hospice approach, which has been so valuable in prioritising and meeting the needs of the younger terminally ill, is shown to be of more limited relevance to the situation of many others who die. Nevertheless, its example may serve as a stimulus for those concerned to develop new approaches to the problems of dying in old age.

The next three chapters (ten, eleven and twelve) consider the role of other forms of institutional provision, more commonly experienced than hospice care by those in the last year of their lives. Chapter ten discusses peoples' experience of hospital care, once again highlighting the needs of the elderly. As shown in the introductory chapter, national statistics reveal changes in the provision and use of hospital care, involving shorter lengths of stay and yet an increasing proportion of deaths occurring within hospitals rather than in peoples' own homes. The effect of these changes is explored in chapter ten.

While provision of hospital care has changed, it was shown in chapter one that there has at the same time been substantial growth in provision of residential and nursing homes places, particularly in the private sector, in the years that separate the two studies. The role of such homes is likely to increase in importance in the future, as the proportion of the population aged 85 and over increases. It is therefore important to understand the circumstances that lead to people entering nursing and residential homes, and to assess the quality of care once there. These matters are covered in chapter eleven.

The final chapter in this part of the book concerns a sector of care that falls between definitions of institutional and community care, and is somewhat neglected in the literature: day centres. It is worth noting that in 1987 hospice day centre provision was a relatively small part of the hospice contribution, with only 58 such centres recorded in England and Wales. By 1993 this had become much more important, with 185 services being in existence (see Table 1.1).

However, day centres or day hospitals provided by local authorities or the NHS generally serve an elderly population not designated as terminally ill, and are much more widespread. They share with hospice facilities the broad aim of enabling people dependent on care in their own homes to stay there, by giving those who care for them at home a break, thereby making entry to more expensive and perhaps less desirable institutional care less likely. In some cases they also aim to ease discharge from hospital to the community by providing rehabilitation facilities. In a climate of concern about public expenditure, coupled with increases in the proportion of the population who are elderly, such provision is likely to assume an increasingly important role. Chapter twelve, written by Graham Farrow who assisted in the later stages of the study, reports on the experiences people had of this form of care.

8 The experience of hospice care

In 1986 a leader in The Lancet stated that "An academic review of hospice services is long overdue". The rapid growth of these services in Britain was described in chapter one (see Table 1.1) so that by 1987 there were 105 in-patient units and 183 home care teams in England and Wales. However, the evaluative effort outside St Christopher's has been slight. Almost all the evaluations of hospice care in Britain have focused on St Christopher's and have, for the most part, been done by Parkes (Parkes 1979a, 1979b, 1980, 1981, Parkes and Parkes 1984, Hinton 1979). An exception is Lunt's (1985) study in Southampton. This situation is in marked contrast to that in America, where a number of studies covering many different hospice sites have been done, the most notable of which is the National Hospice Study (1986).

These studies have been reviewed elsewhere (Seale 1989). Suffice to say that the British studies generally take the form of comparing hospital with hospice experiences using the recollections of relatives several months after the death. Parkes' studies have, on the whole, been encouraging in suggesting that many of the aims of hospice care are being met in St Christopher's. The analysis in this chapter follows an approach similar to that of Parkes, in that relatives and others who knew a sample of people who had died were interviewed some time after the death, and hospice patients and people receiving conventional care are compared, using matched pairs where appropriate. It is the first evaluative study in Britain including in-patient hospice services to cover more than two hospice sites (it covers 14 in-patient hospices), and includes hospice home care as well as in-patient care.

Use of hospice care

The initial random sample of 800 contained 217 people who died of cancer, of whom 14 per cent died in a hospice (institutions were designated hospices if they were listed in the 1987 St Christopher's "Hospice Directory") and 54 per cent died in a hospital. An extra 11 deaths of people who died in hospices were taken from an additional sample of 600 in the same ten areas in order to increase the numbers of people receiving hospice care for the analysis reported in this chapter. Thus, out of the total sample of 1400 randomly selected death registration forms, 41 people, 2.9 per cent, died in a hospice. Attempts have been made by various authors to estimate the numbers of people dying in hospices. These estimates range from 7 per cent of cancer deaths (Rees 1982) to 5 per cent of all deaths (Standing Medical Advisory Committee 1980) and 4 per cent of all deaths (Fry 1983).
However, dying in a hospice is not necessarily an indicator of the total use of hospice services, as people receiving either in-patient or home hospice care may die elsewhere. Excluding the 11 extra hospice deaths and considering the initial random sample of 800 deaths, for whom we got 639 interviews, 6.9 per cent received hospice services in some form, and this included two people who did not die of cancer.

The bulk of this chapter reports the experiences of 45 people who died of cancer and received hospice services, compared to 126 other people who died from cancer.[1] For certain analyses, largely concerning medical procedures where it was felt that the site of cancer might influence the outcome, an analysis of 26 matched pairs who died as in-patients is presented. These pairs are matched for site of cancer and sex, but the hospice patients in the matched pairs are slightly younger than the hospital patients (31 per cent of the hospice deaths were under 65 compared to 8 per cent of the non hospice deaths).

People who received hospice care

People who received hospice care had fewer conditions other than cancer mentioned on the death certificate than those receiving conventional care. Only five hospice patients had other conditions mentioned (11 per cent) whereas of the other people 47 (37 per cent) had other conditions mentioned including 10 per cent who had two. Respiratory and circulatory conditions accounted for most of the these other conditions. Hospice patients were also said to be more likely to have a strong religious faith than people receiving conventional care (49 per cent compared with 23 per cent) and of those who were religious, hospice patients were more likely to be said to have been helped by this faith (80 per cent compared with 63 per cent).

The hospice patients were more likely to have lived in areas south of the Bristol-Wash line (76 per cent did so, compared with 40 per cent of others with cancer) and, on this basis, it might have been expected that their social class might be different. However, although the hospice patients were more likely to come from social classes I, II and III (38 per cent compared to 23 per cent), this difference was not significant. Nor were significant differences found in the types of cancer that the two groups had, home ownership, whether they lived in Metropolitan or County areas, whether they were married, lived alone, or the type of their religious faith.

Out of 23 symptoms asked about, five were experienced significantly more by the hospice patients: pain (93 per cent compared to 80 per cent), sleeplessness (67 per cent compared to 48 per cent), constipation (68 per cent compared to 40 per cent), bedsores (42 per cent compared to 24 per cent) and backache (49 per cent compared to 28 per cent). No symptoms were experienced significantly more by people receiving conventional care.

Concerning the restrictions asked about (see p.82) in each case hospice patients were more likely to experience them, but these differences only reached statistical significance for making a hot drink (63 per cent compared to 41 per cent) and "any other thing" (40 per cent compared to 20 per cent).

So although hospice patients were less likely to suffer from other conditions than cancer, there were slight tendencies for symptoms and restrictions to be reported as having been experienced more frequently. To an extent, this may be due to the sampling method, with the hospice sample weighted towards those needing in-patient care because of the addition of 11 extra in-patient hospice deaths. But the fact that the need for care in the hospice group tended to be greater should be borne in mind when interpreting the results that follow.

Awareness of illness and its consequences

Although the hospice patients were not, according to respondents, significantly more likely to know what was wrong with them, hospice patients were more likely to know that they were going to die. Ninety five per cent of hospice patients were said to have "certainly" or "probably" known this, as opposed to 67 per cent of people receiving conventional care. This contrasts with another British study of awareness comparing hospice with non hospice patients (Gilhooley et al. 1988) which showed no significance difference according to general practitioners' reports. The difference for hospice patients found in the present study may have little to do with hospice practice, as none of the people who knew they were dying had been told so by a hospice doctor or nurse. In fact, as was shown in chapter three, Table 3.5 most of the people in the sample who were said to have known they were likely to die of their illness had guessed this for themselves, without being told by anyone. Of those who were told by someone, hospital doctors were the most likely to be the person who told. No significant difference between hospice patients and people with cancer in conventional care was found in whether they were told they would die by someone, in whether the person who died had asked someone or in whether the respondent had talked with the person who died about their death.

Home nursing[2]

Most (87 per cent) of the hospice patients received visits from a nurse at their home at some stage in their last 12 months, more than those receiving conventional care, 52 per cent of whom were visited in the year (people in nursing homes excluded). Of those who did receive home nursing services, hospice patients were visited more often: 84 per cent had more than 11 visits in the year as opposed to 66 per cent of those in conventional care. This might be expected as, by definition, the hospice group was one receiving services. The higher frequency of symptoms and restrictions in the hospice group (see above) suggests that their need for nursing care may have been greater. This conclusion is supported by the fact that, in spite of receiving less care, the respondents for those in conventional care were equally likely to say that there was not enough nursing help, with 21 per cent of each group saying this.

Respondents were asked in more detail about the types of nurse who helped the most. If more than two types of nurse helped, the two types who helped the most were chosen. This meant that in the hospice sample 25 hospice nurses and 36 district nurses were included. In the conventional care group 61 district nurses were included.

Hospice nurses were more likely than the district nurses of either group to start visiting nearer the end of the illness. Thus 64 per cent of them started visiting a month or less before the death, while this was true of only 33 per cent of all the district nurses. There was no difference in this between the district nurses of the hospice group and those of the other people. There were differences in what the nurses did when visiting. Forty eight per cent of hospice nurses were said to have mainly spent time talking rather than providing practical care when they visited, as opposed to 17 per cent of district nurses.

Most (85 per cent) of the nurses were said to have had enough time to do the things they did rather than hurrying, and there was no difference between the types of nurse in this. However, respondents said that they would have liked 17 per cent of the district nurses to have done more than they did, and this was said of none of the hospice nurses. Hospice nurses were perceived as having given more reassurance and support than district nurses, and the same is true of district nurses of hospice patients compared to district nurses of people receiving conventional care, as Table 8.1 shows.

Table 8.1
Respondents' views about the degree of reassurance and support provided by domiciliary nurses

	Hospice patients		Non Hospice patients
	Hospice Nurses	District Nurses	District Nurses
Would you say (the nurses) gave (the patient):	%	%	%
A lot of reassurance and support	92	69	42
Some reassurance and support	8	31	45
or Hardly any reassurance and support?	0	0	13
Number of people (100%)	24	36	53

This difference may reflect the quality of advice offered by the nurses, as the nurses of hospice patients (whether they were district or hospice nurses) were more likely to be seen as offering "very helpful" as opposed to "fairly helpful" advice (91 per cent compared with 58 per cent of the nurses of people receiving conventional care). Overall, the nursing help and care of hospice patients was rated more highly than that of others. Seventy one per cent of the nursing episodes of hospice patients were said to have involved "excellent" care, 24 per cent "good" care and 5 per cent fair or poor care. Only 48 per cent of the nurses of the conventional care group were judged excellent, 36 per cent good and 16 per cent fair or poor.

Clearly hospice home care nurses played a different role from district nurses. The results support those of Ward (1985) who showed that such nurses are more likely to act in an advisory and supportive capacity, and are less likely to get involved in the day to day practical tasks of nursing care. To some extent, the extra care that these nurses gave may have taken some pressure off the district nurses visiting the same patients, allowing them the time to provide a greater degree of reassurance and support than district nurses working on their own. At any rate, the value placed on the services of specialist home nursing by respondents is clearly very great.

In-patient care

Saunders (1978, Saunders and Baines 1983) has expressed her belief in the importance of involving the family in the care of their dying relatives, and support for families in keeping people at home for as long as possible is the avowed aim of many hospice practitioners. Fourteen different in-patient hospices were represented in the achieved sample and 33 people dying of cancer were in-patients in these hospices. Excluding the extra in-patient hospice deaths, cancer patients receiving significant amounts of hospice services were no less likely to die as in-patients than those receiving conventional care. When the length of final stay was compared for those who died as in-patients, people dying in hospices spent less time there on final admission compared to people dying in hospitals: 41 per cent of hospice patients spent less than a week there, as opposed to 20 per cent of hospital patients, and this difference was maintained in the sample of pairs matched for site of cancer (40 per cent and 15 per cent). However, the overall length of time spent as an in-patient anywhere in the last 12 months of life was not significantly different, in spite of the greater provision of home nursing services for the hospice group.

A key principle of palliative medical care is that prolonging life at the expense of unnecessary suffering should be avoided where possible (Saunders 1978, Saunders and Baines 1983). Whether the treatments received by either group of people were palliative in this sense is difficult to judge in the absence of other medical data. However the data do indicate that the hospice group experienced fewer medical interventions of a curative and investigative nature as they approached death.

Considering the whole of the last 12 months of life of people who died as in-patients, people in the hospice group were less likely to have an operation (15 per cent of the hospice group had one, as opposed to 31 per cent of the others). When the final admissions of those dying as in-patients were considered, the divergence between the groups for medical procedures became more extreme. People receiving conventional care who died in hospital were significantly more likely to have an operation on their last admission (30 per cent) than were people who died in hospices, none of whom had operations. This difference remained significant for the 26 matched pairs (31 per cent compared with none). Of those who had operations, 76 per cent involved a curative or investigative purpose rather than being purely for palliative symptom relief. All the operations on people in the matched pairs were done for curative or investigative reasons. People in the conventional care group who died in hospital were more likely to be admitted for curative or investigative reasons than were people who died in hospices, when reasons for the final admission were considered. Thus all but one of the hospice group were said to have been admitted solely for terminal care or symptom relief at this stage, as opposed to only a third of the people receiving conventional care. For matched pairs the figures were 95 per cent of the hospice group and 29 per cent of the conventional care group.

Practitioners of palliative medical care also emphasise the importance of symptom relief in terminal cancer, particularly pain (Saunders 1978, Saunders and Baines 1983). Respondents were asked to comment in detail about the care received for pain, breathlessness and nausea. Only for pain were the numbers suffering the symptom great enough for significance testing. Answers were compared for final admissions that ended in death, and for the matched pairs. For the first comparison, all 11 hospice patients suffering pain had it relieved completely all or some of the time, but only 28 of the 41 people receiving conventional care (68 per cent) were said to have been relieved to this extent. The difference was maintained for matched pairs (ten out of ten hospice patients and ten out of 15 people receiving conventional care).

Hospice principles also involve the provision of a welcoming atmosphere for visitors, so that they can play a part in looking after their dying relatives. Respondents who visited the people during the final admission were asked if they had helped in their care. No significant difference between hospital and hospice visitors was found. They were also asked whether they had been treated very or fairly kindly, indifferently or with hostility by staff during visits. No respondents recorded the last option, but hospice respondents all recorded "very kindly" as compared with 77 per cent of hospital respondents.

Hospital patients were more likely to have a room to themselves "some of the time" (34 per cent compared with 4 per cent) rather than "all the time" or "not at all", perhaps reflecting a policy of moving patients to a single room when near to death. For those who were never in a single room, it was said for 17 per cent that they would have preferred one, with no significant difference between hospice and hospital patients. Hospice patients were significantly more likely to be judged to have been in a "very peaceful and quiet" room at the time of death (87 per cent compared with 49 per cent).

Finally, overall ratings of care provided by medical and nursing staff were asked for. Firstly, respondents were asked if they felt doctors had been able and willing to give the time to the dying person that she or he needed. Of the 94 who gave a definite reply to this question, the six who said "no" were all relatives of hospital patients (numbers were too low for significance testing). Respondents were then asked to rate the care received from doctors and that received from nurses and other staff. Results are shown in Table 8.2 and Table 8.3 and show that both doctors' and nurses' care was more likely to be rated as excellent by respondents for the hospice group.

Table 8.2
Respondents' views of the care from doctors during in-patient stays

Would you describe the different aspects of care (the patient) got from the doctor as:	Hospice %	Hospital %
Excellent	91	40
Good	9	49
Fair	0	7
or Poor?	0	4
Number of people (100%)	22	77

Table 8.3
Respondents' views about nursing care during in-patient stays

What about the nurses and other staff there? Do you think the care (the patient) got from them was:	Hospice %	Hospital %
Excellent	96	57
Good	4	33
Fair	0	9
or Poor?	0	1
Number of people (100%)	24	79

At the time of death

Bowling (1983) has argued that the trend towards hospitalisation at the time of death has adverse consequences: more people die alone or without their relatives and friends, and this means that the pain of bereavement for those unable to say "goodbye" is worse. It was shown earlier that dying as an in-patient was no more likely for either the hospice or conventional care group. The data also show that dissatisfaction with the site of death, whether at home or in hospital, was no different. This contrasts with the findings of the United States National Hospice Study (1986) which found that carers of hospice patients were more satisfied with the site of death. Dying alone was not significantly more likely for either group, nor was there a significant difference in whether respondents who had not been present would have liked to have been.

Cathcart (1988) has reviewed the sparse evidence that exists to support a widely held view that seeing the body after death helps with the grieving process, concluding that seeing the body is beneficial, though reluctance to do so should always be respected. Sixty four per cent of respondents saw the body after death, and there was no significant difference between the hospice and conventional care groups.

The only significant difference between the two groups in what happened at the time of death concerned the way in which respondents for people who died as in-patients felt they had been treated at this time by staff. Supporting respondents' positive ratings of the quality of care from doctors and nurses in hospices, respondents for the hospice group were more likely to say that staff had been "very kind and understanding" as opposed to "fairly" or "not" than were the conventional care group (100 per cent compared to 82 per cent).

After the death

Respondents were asked a number of questions about who they had seen and talked to about their feelings since the death, and how well they had adjusted to life without the person who had died. Answers were analyzed both for all respondents and for spouses only.

Respondents for the hospice group were more likely than the others to be visited by a nurse at home after the death (30 per cent were visited, compared to 16 per cent), but this difference was not significant when spouses only were considered. Visits at home from a number of other professionals, visits by the respondent to the general practitioner, wanting a visit from someone or wanting to talk to someone about their feelings were not significantly different between the groups.

Symptoms related to bereavement, such as sleeplessness, nerves and depression and loss of appetite, were not reported significantly more by either group except when spouses alone were considered, where spouses of the hospice group were less likely to report sleeplessness (46 per cent compared to 75 per cent).

Respondents were also asked about loneliness, whether they could look forward to things in the way they used to, whether they felt they had come to terms with the death, how much they missed the person who had died and how things were going for them generally. Some of the items were taken from Bowling and Cartwright's (1982) study of the elderly widowed, and were designed to assess how well people adjusted to bereavement. On none of these questions was there a significant difference between respondents for the hospice group and others. However, of those who reported loneliness, hospice respondents were significantly more likely to say that they would get over it soon rather than it being a big problem (69 per cent compared with 35 per cent). This difference remained when spouses only were considered (75 per cent compared with 28 per cent).

Conclusion

As an evaluation of hospice care, this analysis is limited because there was no random allocation to either group. The hospice group had fewer conditions other than cancer recorded on their death certificates, had more symptoms and restrictions and tended to be more religious. All of these things might have influenced the outcome measures. Random allocation is difficult to achieve in health services research for practical and ethical reasons, and the only other study in this field that practised random allocation (Kane et al. 1984) failed to separate the treatment and control groups adequately (Mahoney 1986, Higginson and McCarthy 1989, Seale 1989). The present study is more like that of Parkes and Parkes' (1984) evaluation of St Christopher's hospice, where control of extraneous variables was achieved to some extent (and where appropriate) by matching pairs on relevant variables.

A further consideration is the validity of using relatives' accounts rather than those of the people who died. The widespread use of this method in evaluations of hospice care has been questioned, for example, by Ahmedzai et al. (1988). Our review of the literature on the use of proxy respondents in studies of the terminally ill (Cartwright and Seale 1990) showed areas of disagreement between studies on the direction and extent of differences. Our own study of 34 pairs of people with terminal cancer and their relatives showed that relatives tended to be more critical of the quality of care, and to report more symptoms than the people who died (Cartwright and Seale 1990). This is partly because dying people cannot all be interviewed on the day they die, and so were reporting on a different time period from relatives. The mental confusion of some people can also distort accounts; nor can dying people report on events at or after their deaths. A full report of this methodological study, and data relevant to the related issue of congruence between relatives' and health care professionals' accounts is provided in Cartwright and Seale (1990).

The hospice group in this study were somewhat more likely to know that they would die of their disease, although this may have been because they were people who conveyed that they were ready to cope with the knowledge to a greater extent than the people in conventional care. In this area, it might be argued that the hospice movement as a whole deserves to be evaluated not just in terms of the immediate effect of specific services on patients receiving them, but in terms of its influence on terminal care in general. In chapter three it was shown that people with terminal cancer were more likely in 1987 than in 1969 to know that they would die and that this was largely because hospital doctors had become more inclined to tell them. This shift towards openness in communication with dying people may have to do with the approach advocated by hospice practitioners.

What the analysis reveals beyond question, however, is that the process of hospice care, in both in-patient and home care settings, was rather different from conventional care and that hospice care was, in many respects, seen as valuable. Ward's (1985) study describing the work of hospice home care teams is supported by the current study. Hospice home care nurses were less involved in practical aspects of care and more in providing advice and support. It is perhaps unfair to compare them with district nurses who had a different role, but an important finding was that hospice home nursing care combined with district nursing care was more likely to be seen as having providing a lot of reassurance and support and more likely to have provided excellent help and care than district nursing alone.

The less interventionist approach of medical staff, and the caring and supportive atmosphere provided for respondents by hospice staff appear to have been similarly appreciated. Attention to symptom control appears to have paid off, resulting in better pain control in hospices. However, caution should be exercised in concluding too much from the findings about in-patient care as many aspects of patients' experiences may have been determined by medical differences between the groups which were only crudely controlled for by matching for site of cancer and sex.

The experience of respondents at the time of death and in bereavement afterwards did not show as many differences between the groups as was the case in care before the death. But it may be concluded from this analysis that, given the sort of people who do, in practice, enter hospice care, satisfaction with that care reported by respondents after the death is high, and generally higher than that of respondents for people receiving conventional care.

Notes

1. The hospice group excludes the two non cancer deaths receiving hospice services. Hospice care for the remaining 49 consisted of 24 who received in-patient hospice care only (some of these were visited by District Nurses), nine who received in-patient hospice care and hospice home care, and 16 who received hospice home care only. Four of those receiving hospice home care only had minimal amounts (for example, one visit from a Marie Curie night sitter) and have been excluded from the analyses reported here except in certain analyses covering home nursing services.

2. The four people who received minimal amounts of hospice home care (see note 1) are included in the analysis for this section, bringing the hospice group up to 49. This is because the purpose of much of the analysis is to establish whether nursing care was of an adequate amount, and it would make no sense to exclude hospice cases with small amounts of care if a valid comparison of hospice versus people receiving conventional care is to be achieved.

9 Hospices in context

Hospices are, largely, specialist terminal care services, focusing on cancer patients. Yet those centrally involved in the development of these services have argued that their philosophy of terminal care should not be confined to cancer alone. Thus Saunders and Baines (1983) state that:

> ...many of the symptoms to be treated and much of the general management will be relevant to other situations... Terminal care should not only be a part of oncology but of geriatric medicine, neurology, general practice and throughout medicine.

Elsewhere Saunders (1978) has referred to developments taking place in hospice provision to include "a mixed group of patients", including disorders other than cancer, and the care of elderly people without malignant disease. However, as the last chapter showed, this type of provision is as yet of limited size in Britain.

Blackburn (1989) in a study of 27 elderly men dying on a geriatric ward concluded that these patients needed a different type of terminal care from younger people with cancer. Communication difficulties were more frequent with the elderly group, and the diagnosis of dying was more difficult and occurred closer to the time of death. He noted the relative absence of family visitors for his sample. Wilson et al. (1987) present a palliative approach to the treatment of terminally ill elderly people which stresses the long term nature of the problem: the median length of stay on long term wards in Wilson's sample was nine months.

This chapter for the most part presents a comparison of those in the sample who died of cancer with people dying of other conditions in an attempt to further the debate about the applicability of the hospice approach to conditions other than cancer.

Demographic characteristics and social support

Cancer, accounting for 27 per cent of the deaths in the sample of 800, was just about equally spread between males and females, with 52 per cent of people dying from cancer being male. Perhaps the most important feature of death from cancer in predicting levels of social support as well as many other aspects of the experience of people with terminal cancer is the age at death. People dying from cancer were younger, on the whole, than people dying from other conditions, as is demonstrated in Table 9.1, which uses information from the 800 death certificates chosen for the sample.

The relative youth of people dying from cancer meant that their family composition tended to be different from that of others. Table 9.2 presents data illustrating this for the 639 people for whom we obtained interviews. This shows that people who did not die of cancer were more likely to be widowed and to be women, and this was largely due to the preponderance of the elderly in the non cancer group. In fact 63 per cent of people dying from cancer were survived by a spouse, while this was true for only 39 per cent of others. Not only were people with cancer more likely to have siblings alive, they were also more likely to have children alive. People dying of conditions other than cancer were more likely to have no immediate family (12 per cent of them, compared to 4 per cent of people with cancer). People living alone, and those in nursing or residential homes, were also more common in the non cancer group.

Symptoms and restrictions

The people who died from cancer in the sample were said to have been more likely than others to have suffered from a number of symptoms and to have experienced restriction in their daily activities at some stage in the last 12 months of life. However, within this broad generalisation there were exceptions, and the picture is modified when duration and intensity are considered. Table 9.3 shows the symptoms reported for people with cancer compared with others, separately presented by age.

Pain in people with cancer was not only more common, but was reported to be more distressing where it did occur, compared to pain in people who did not have cancer. Thus 60 per cent of those with cancer suffering pain were said to have found it "very distressing" whereas this was true of 48 per cent of others experiencing pain. Significant differences in the degree of distress for people with cancer were also found for loss of appetite, constipation, trouble with breathing, nausea and vomiting and sleeplessness, although the reported duration of symptoms for the people with cancer

Table 9.1
Proportion of deaths from cancer, by age

	Age				
	15-54	55-64	65-74	75-84	85+
Per cent cancer	35%	34%	41%	23%	11%
Number of deaths (=100%)	78	101	185	264	172

Table 9.2
Sex, family and place of residence by cause of death and age

	Cancer			Non cancer		
	Under 75	Over 75	All ages	Under 75	Over 75	All ages
	%	%	%	%	%	%
Women	44	48	45	34*	69*	55*
Widowed	13	48	25	19	57*	43*
No siblings alive	19	46	28	19	52	39*
No child alive	18	21	19	27*	36*	33*
Stayed in nursing/ old peoples' home in last 12 months	4	14	7	7	42*	29*
Living alone	14	28	18	23	33	29*
Total number of deaths (=100%)	110	58	168	179	292	471

*Indicates a statistically significant difference with the same age cancer group ($p < 0.05$, chi square statistic)

Table 9.3
Symptoms reported as experienced in the last 12 months of life in a sample of 639 adults by cause of death and age

	Cancer			Non cancer		
	Under 75	Over 75	All ages	Under 75	Over 75	All ages
	%	%	%	%	%	%
Pain	88	75	84	67*	68	67*
Trouble with breathing	51	40	47	50	49	49
Vomiting or feeling sick	51	52	51	26*	27*	27*
Drowsiness	57	59	58	34*	43*	39*
Sleeplessness	57	39	51	32*	39	36*
Dry mouth/thirst	52	41	48	25*	27*	27*
Mental confusion	30	39	33	21	49	38
Depression	39	38	38	37	35	36
Loss of appetite	77	58	71	29*	43*	38*
Difficulty in swallowing	40	35	38	15*	18*	17*
Constipation	49	44	47	25*	37	32*
Persistent cough	32	23	29	29	12*	18*
Dizziness	21	43	29	24	35	30
Dribbling	13	9	11	10	16	14
Bad temper	14	23	17	27*	24	25*
Bedsores	33	17	28	7*	18	14*
Loss of bladder control	32	46	37	15*	43	33
Loss of bowel control	25	26	25	11*	28	22
Unpleasant smell	18	20	19	9*	15	13
Difficulty seeing (with spectacles)	12	28	18	14	34*	27*
Difficulty hearing	13	39	22	13	41*	31*
Backache	36	29	34	30	29	30
Other	36	31	34	31	36	34
Total number of deaths (=100%)	110	58	168	179	292	471

*Indicates a statistically significant difference with the same age cancer group ($p < 0.05$, chi square statistic)

was not usually as great. In particular, long term pain (where the person was reported to have had it for a year or more) was reported less commonly for people with cancer than others (41 per cent compared with 66 per cent) and was particularly common in stroke (73 per cent) and respiratory disease (83 per cent). Breathing trouble and nausea and vomiting were more likely to be reported as long term in people without cancer who had the symptoms (60 per cent compared with 42 per cent for breathing trouble; 42 per cent compared with 19 per cent for nausea and vomiting). Mental confusion followed the same pattern: in people without cancer this was much more likely to be reported as a long term problem (65 per cent compared with 21 per cent). Significant differences for duration between cancer patients and others were also found for loss of appetite, difficulty swallowing, constipation, drowsiness and sleeplessness.

Table 9.4
Restrictions experienced at home by a sample of adults in the last 12 months of life, by age and cause[a]

	Cancer			Non cancer		
	Under 75	Over 75	All ages	Under 75	Over 75	All ages
	%	%	%	%	%	%
Needed help with:						
Get in/out bath/shower	64	61	63	32*	67	55
Dress/undress	53	36	48	20*	44	35*
Go to toilet	51	33	45	16*	35	28*
Wash (and shave)	45	33	41	16*	37	29*
Feed him/herself	24	18	22	7*	22	17
Cut own toenails	63	72	66	30*	77	60
Make hot drink	54	35	48	20*	47	37*
Help at night	55	35	49	23*	41	34*
Any other thing	30	20	26	18*	33	27
At least one of the above	81	74	79	40*	78	65*
Total number of deaths (=100%)	110	55	165	154	284	438

*Indicates a statistically significant difference with the same age cancer group ($p < 0.05$, chi square statistic)

[a] Excludes sudden death under 65 and those in hospital for 12 months before death

The restrictions reported are presented in Table 9.4, separately for age and cause of death. It will be seen that, when the younger groups are compared, restrictions of every sort were more likely to have been experienced by people with cancer. In contrast, Table 9.5 presents the picture for *long term* restriction, which shows that this was reported more commonly for people dying from causes other than cancer. This was largely due to the much higher incidence of long term restriction in the elderly non cancer group.

Table 9.5
Experience of long term restriction[a], by age and cause[b]

	Cancer			Non cancer		
	Under 75	Over 75	All ages	Under 75	Over 75	All ages
	%	%	%	%	%	%
Needed help with:						
Get in/out bath/shower	13	20	15	17	50*	38*
Dress/undress	10	2	7	11	26*	21*
Go to toilet	6	2	5	7	17*	14*
Wash (and shave)	4	2	3	6	19*	15*
Feed him/herself	2	0	1	3	8*	6*
Cut own toenails	22	44	29	20	63*	47*
Make hot drink	13	10	12	10	31*	24*
Help at night	7	4	6	12	24*	20*
Any other thing	7	6	6	9	22*	17*
At least one of the above	20	29	23	22	60*	46*
Total number of deaths (=100%)	110	55	165	154	284	438

*Indicates a statistically significant difference with the same age cancer group ($p < 0.05$, chi square statistic)

[a] ie: had restriction for a year or more

[b] Excludes sudden death under 65 and those in hospital all year

The picture of cancer which emerges, then, is of a disease that tends to produce a number of symptoms that are intensely distressing, such as pain, breathlessness and vomiting, but which are of relatively short duration. In conditions other than cancer, degenerating sight and hearing and long term mental confusion are problems, particularly in the elderly. Long term restrictions and consequent dependency are also more a feature of the elderly person not suffering from cancer, although cancer is associated with a high incidence of short term restriction.

Sources of help

Informal care

Differences in the sources of help for people with cancer compared to others reflected the differences in household and family composition described earlier. Thus, for those who experienced restrictions at some stage in their last 12 months, help with these was given by a relative or friend to 94 per cent of people with cancer, but only 67 per cent of those without cancer. People without cancer were more likely to get help from residential staff (38 per cent, compared with 8 per cent of people with cancer) and from a chiropodist (53 per cent compared to 20 per cent). Respondents who had taken part in caring for the person who died were asked a number of questions about the effect of this on their lives. The response of those caring for people with cancer suggest that the relatively rapid onset of distressing symptoms and restrictions was more disruptive of carers' lives, albeit over a shorter time period, than for those helping people with other conditions. Relatives who had cared for people with cancer were more likely to report that they gave up visiting friends (52 per cent compared with 31 per cent), going out to social activities (55 per cent compared with 30 per cent) and entertaining people at home (41 per cent compared with 23 per cent).

The restriction on the social lives of those caring for those who did not have cancer may have been equally great, but the care was likely to have been needed over a longer period, and the impact on the carers' lives would have been more gradual. Differences in the social contacts of carers of people who do not have cancer are also suggested by the finding that these people were more likely to say they gave up or did less looking after someone else as a result of looking after the person who died (16 per cent compared with 8 per cent).

Formal provision

Frequent contacts over a relatively short period characterise the pattern of domiciliary care for those who died from cancer. This reflects the pattern of shorter term but more intense symptoms and restrictions found in the cancer group. People with cancer were more likely to be reported as receiving visits from a nurse at their home during their last 12 months (63 per cent compared with 30 per cent). Of those who received help from district nurses, long term help (a year or more) was more common in people without cancer (39 per cent compared with 18 per cent). People with cancer, on the other hand, were reported as more likely to receive intensive district nursing care (defined as visits at least once a day [52 per cent compared with 32 per cent]).

Excluding people in hospital for a year or more before death and people under 65 who died suddenly, people with cancer were reported to have consulted a general practitioner more frequently than others: 30 per cent consulted more than 20 times, compared to only 16 per cent of others. People with cancer were also more likely to receive a home visit from a general practitioner (89 per cent compared with 80 per cent) and were more likely to be visited at night (36 per cent compared with 24 per cent).

Respondents' evaluations of the quality of care suggest that these differences in the pattern of visiting were an appropriate response to differing patterns of need. When asked to judge whether nursing help had been needed but not provided very few said that this was the case (5 per cent overall) and no difference was found between those with cancer and those who did not have cancer. Of those receiving help from nurses visiting the home, respondents in each group were equally likely to be satisfied with the amount of help. No difference was evident in respondents' ratings of the quality of care from the general practitioner.

The amount of in-patient care was also different for the two groups. People with cancer were more likely to enter a hospital or hospice during the last 12 months of life (95 per cent compared with 70 per cent) and, of those who did enter, people with cancer were more likely to be in more than one (38 per cent compared with 21 per cent). Measures of satisfaction with nursing and medical care in hospital again showed no significant difference between respondents for cancer patients and others.

Knowledge about illness and death

One of the most significant aspects of the hospice approach to terminal care is that of communication with people and their families about illness and death. In this area, again, there were differences reported between the cancer group and others. People dying from cancer were said to be more likely to know what was wrong with them, and that they would die from it, than people dying from other conditions. Table 9.6 shows reported awareness of diagnosis and prognosis in both the people who died and in respondents, with people who died suddenly or with no evident illness excluded from the figures.[1]

The length of time over which respondents knew the person would die was also greater for people with cancer. Of those respondents for those without cancer who had known the person would die, 33 per cent knew this for less than a week before death, this being true of only 10 per cent of cancer deaths. While the proportion of those respondents knowing for more than a year ahead that death would occur was similar (20 per cent and 19 per cent), over half (52 per cent) of the respondents for people with cancer knew the person would die between one month and one year beforehand. This was true of only 23 per cent of the others who had forewarning. Blackburn's

Table 9.6
Knowledge of diagnosis and awareness of likely death, by age and cause[a]

	Cancer			Non cancer		
	Under 75 %	Over 75 %	All ages %	Under 75 %	Over 75 %	All ages %
Diagnosis						
Deceased knew	86	74	82	81	60*	67*
Respondent knew	86	79	84	82	78	79
Would certainly/probably die						
Deceased knew	75	74	75	53*	54*	54*
Respondent knew	90	89	90	48*	53*	51*
Total number of deaths (=100%)	110	57	167	111	243	354

*Indicates a statistically significant difference with the same age cancer group (p < 0.05, chi square statistic)

[a]Sudden deaths and deaths of people with no apparent illness or incapacity excluded

(1989) comment that "The diagnosis of dying...is more difficult in the absence of neoplasia..." is supported by these data.

The degree to which respondents accepted the death was influenced both by the age of the deceased and the cause of death. As Table 9.7 shows,[2] respondents for people with cancer were more likely to feel (taking illness into account) that the person had died at the best time, and this was particularly marked in the older groups. For those over 75, respondents for people who did not have cancer were significantly more likely to feel that earlier would have been better. This probably reflects the burden of long term disability and dependence that were suffered by people who did not have cancer in their final year of life. The intensity of suffering for those with cancer compared to others may have led many respondents to feel that death was a welcome release.

Table 9.7
Views about the time of death, by cause and age (excluding sudden deaths)

Looking back now, and taking .....'s illness into account, do you think he/she died at the best time, or would it have been better if he/she had died earlier or later?

	Cancer			Non cancer		
	Under 75	Over 75	All ages	Under 75	Over 75	All ages
	%	%	%	%	%	%
Died at best time	62	83	70	50	63*	59*
Better earlier	23	13	19	20	28*	26
Better later	15	4	11	30*	9	15
Total number of deaths (=100%)	88	47	135	86	213	299

*Indicates a statistically significant difference with the same age cancer group ($p < 0.05$, chi square statistic)

Conclusion

This chapter has shown that people who die from cancer are different in many of the key variables that determine treatment and care. The incidence, duration, intensity and type of symptoms follow a different pattern in cancer compared to other illnesses. Pain is more likely to be a problem and is more intense when it does occur. The same is true of a number of other symptoms, the control of which has been the focus of a great deal of valuable effort by hospice practitioners. Long term mental confusion and disability, as well as other symptoms related to age, are more common in those without cancer.

In fact, age appears to be the crucial factor in determining how people with cancer are different. Age not only determines to a large extent physical ailments and restrictions, but also the level of support that can be expected from families. People aged 75 and over who do not die from cancer are more likely to have outlasted their spouses, their brothers and sisters, and even their children. They are predominantly women and many live alone or in residential care. The care of those with cancer tends to be of shorter duration and of greater intensity, judging by the pattern of informal care, nursing visits, general practitioner care and hospital admissions. The fact that satisfaction with the quality of professional care showed no significant differences suggests that the different pattern of care is appropriate, and that needs are being met to an equal degree in both groups.

Thus the medical and nursing needs of people with cancer fit the pattern of care provided by hospices. The emphasis on family involvement and support is clearly more appropriate in cancer because people with cancer are more likely to have families. The service provided by specialist home care teams, emphasising emotional support and advice rather than practical nursing tasks (Ward 1985), is more appropriate with cancer, as the cancer patient is more likely to have an informal carer. That carer is more likely to face unfamiliar tasks, as the disease lasts a shorter time and is more intense, placing a rapidly increasing burden on the carer who will have had relatively little time to adapt to it.

The bereavement services set up by many hospices are also more appropriate in the case of cancer, since the family composition of people dying with cancer means that a bereaved person closely related to the deceased is more likely to be present. In causes of death other than cancer, even where relatives are present, the needs in bereavement support are likely to be different. Sudden deaths of younger people clearly present their own problems, and the chapter has shown that death in the younger person without cancer was least likely to be seen as having occurred at the right time. For the elderly person without cancer a significant number of respondents felt death would, ideally, have come sooner. Grief in these circumstances may be less intensely focused on the actual bereavement, and more on the distress of coping with long term dependency.

Perhaps the second most crucial factor after age in deciding how hospice principles might apply to people without cancer is the relative ease with which a terminal phase can be distinguished in cancer. Blackburn's (1989) point that the diagnosis of dying is more difficult in the elderly is fully supported by the data. It is of interest to note that Brechling and Kuhn (1989) in their attempt to provide hospice style care for people with dementia, found it hard to select people with a prognosis of less than six months as prediction of death was very difficult. The communication issues which have been seen as so important by those working in hospices are usually different when cancer is not present. The moment at which death can be predicted with certainty, if the moment occurs at all, is generally closer to the actual event. Telling or not telling that death is likely to occur is less of an issue, as medical uncertainty may often be coupled with the presence of long term mental confusion and the absence of relatives to whom news can be given.

The hospice philosophy has been to eschew "heroic" medical endeavours designed to prolong life at all costs. Yet heroism of a different nature is present in the hospice approach to terminal cancer care: that in which dramatic moments of truth are reached and confronted, where intensely distressing physical suffering is controlled, and where death and dying is attended by an audience of grieving relatives. None of these things may apply to the same extent in the care of elderly people without cancer, whose family composition and physical needs suggest that a different approach is needed, albeit one that, as in good hospice care, respects people's autonomy and dignity.

Notes

1. The figures in Table 9.6 differ from those in Table 2.6 because the later table includes respondents who were not relatives or close friends. These respondents had to be excluded in the earlier table in order to make comparisons with the 1969 study.

2. Table 9.7 excludes respondents who said they did not know the answer to the question, or gave a reply that did not fit the categories given in the table. This explains the differences with percentages reported in chapters 5 and 6 for this question.

10 Hospitals

In chapter one it was shown that most people in 1987 (64 per cent) died in hospitals. The 1969 study estimated that between a quarter and three tenths of hospital bed days were taken up by people who would be dead within 12 months. Clearly hospitals play a role in the care of many people before their death, and caring for people in the year before they die is a substantial part of hospital work. This chapter is about the extent of hospital or hospice care in the last 12 months of people's lives, the characteristics of people who use the hospital service during this time, changes between 1969 and 1987, and the views of relatives and others about the appropriateness of hospital care for the people who died. Since most people who die are aged 65 or more (80% in 1987 [OPCS 1987]), the focus is on the care of older people.

The death registration forms for the sample of deaths indicated that 58 per cent died in a hospital or hospice with a further two per cent being dead on arrival at hospital. Interview data suggested that of these 60 per cent (who would be recorded in official statistics as dying in a hospital or other institution for the care of the sick), 46 per cent died in a hospital ward and four per cent in a hospice, but six per cent probably died before they reached the hospital and four per cent in an accident and emergency department.

But many more received some care in a hospital or hospice during the year before they died: 76 per cent of all those who died. The estimated average number of admissions was 1.49 (1.44 to hospital, 0.05 to a hospice). Those who were in a hospital or hospice at all were often admitted more than once; in fact an average of two times. The great majority, 97 per cent, of the hospital admissions were under the NHS compared with less than half, 43 per cent, of the admissions to hospices.

The length of time people had been in any hospital or hospice during the last year of their lives is shown in Table 10.1. Two per cent spent all of the last year of their lives in a hospital, another two per cent most of it. A more typical pattern, for 45 per cent, was to spend a relatively short period (less than one month) in a hospital or hospice.

An analysis by age at death showed that people dying at 85 or more were the least likely to have spent any of the last year of their lives in a hospital or hospice: only 63 per cent of them had done so compared with 79 per cent of people dying at younger ages. Henderson et al. (1990) report a similar finding. As was shown in chapter seven, comparatively few of those who were 85 or over had died in a hospital or hospice: 44 per cent compared with 57 per cent of younger people. There were no other marked differences or trends with age. The differences between those aged 85 or more and the others are more notable in that the proportion dying from a cerebrovascular accident increased from none of those aged under 55 to 19 per cent of those aged 75 or more (the proportions were similar for those aged 75-84 and 85+) and, as Table 10.2 shows, those dying from cerebrovascular accident were comparatively high users of the hospital service.

The reason why people aged 85 or more were less likely to spend much of the last year of their lives in hospital is probably that 37 per cent of them spent all the last year of their life in a residential or nursing home and a further 19 per cent spent some of that time in one. People who had lived in an old people's home were less likely than others who died to have gone into a hospital or hospice during the last year of their lives, 62 per cent compared with 81 per cent, or to die in one, 38 per cent compared with 59 per cent.

Table 10.1
Age at death and use of hospital or hospice service

Time spent in hospital or hospice in last 12 months of life	<45 %	45-54 %	55-64 %	65-74 %	75-84 %	85+ %	All %
None	27	28	22	19	20	37	24
Less than a week	14	10	24	17	17	13	17
1 week < 1 month	27	28	32	31	30	21	28
1 month < 3 months	18	26	15	25	23	19	22
3 months or longer	14	8	7	8	10	10	9
Died in a hospital or hospice (%)	52	46	44	54	66	44	54
Number of deaths (=100%)	23	39	80	147	203	147	639

Table 10.2
Cause of death and use of hospital or hospice service

Time spent in hospital or hospice in last year of life	Cause of death						
	1 %	2 %	3 %	4 %	5 %	6 %	7 %
None	5	38	20	37	38	52	19
Less than a week	15	18	16	28	14	19	9
1 week < 1 month	35	25	28	22	23	18	29
1 month < 3 months	36	17	19	7	17	7	22
3 months or more	9	2	17	6	8	4	21
Died in:							
a hospital (%)	52	36	72	47	45	43	61
a hospice (%)	14	-	-	-	-	-	-
Number of deaths (=100%)	168	177	88	47	49	30	80

1 Neoplasm
2 Ischaemic heart disease
3 Cerebrovascular accident
4 Other circulatory
5 Respiratory
6 Injury
7 Other

Nearly all, 95 per cent, of those dying of cancer spent some of the last 12 months in a hospital or hospice and they were the only ones to die in a hospice. Although the duration of symptoms experienced by those dying of cancer was not usually as long as those for people dying of other causes, a comparatively high proportion, 45 per cent, of those dying of cancer spent a month or more in a hospital or hospice. This may be partly because the symptoms of people with cancer tended to be rather more distressing and to need more nursing or medical care.

If availability of care in the community was a factor in determining hospital admission it might be expected that those who normally lived alone would be high users of the hospital service and the married low users (Butler and Morgan 1977). In practice this did not happen. Those living alone made no more use of the hospital service than those living with others, and although they were less likely to die in their own homes (22 per cent compared with 32 per cent) this was because more of them died in residential or nursing homes (13 per cent compared with one per cent). The married were *more* likely to have been in hospital or hospice in the last year of their lives than the never or previously married (82 per cent compared with 70 per cent). This seems to be because married people who die are comparatively young so more of them die of cancer (36 per cent compared with 18 per cent). However, even when cancer deaths are excluded a higher proportion of the married died in hospital (55 per cent compared with 45 per cent). This again seemed to be because more of the single or previously married died in residential homes 26 per cent compared with 3 per cent of the married, and because married people were comparatively frequently admitted to hospital very shortly before their death. Among those who died in hospital of diseases other than cancer 49 per cent of the married, 31 per cent of the others, were admitted less than a week before they died.

Women were no more or less likely than men to die in a hospital or hospice or to be admitted to one in the last year of their lives. They were less likely to die in their own homes, 20 per cent compared with 30 per cent for men, and more likely to die in a residential home, 21 per cent compared with 4 per cent.

Rough estimates from the data suggest that the people who died spent an average of 38 days in NHS hospitals or hospices in the year before their death, and when multiplied by the total number of deaths this represents approximately 22 per cent of all occupied NHS hospital bed days in 1986 (DoH 1988). This compares with an estimate of between 25 per cent and 30 per cent in 1969, and suggests that there has been a fall in the proportion of hospital resources spent on the care of people who would soon be dead. A probable reason for this change is the increase in residential homes. Other changes between the two studies were a 50 per cent rise in the number of hospital admissions, a much smaller increase in the proportion dying in hospital, and therefore an increase in the number of discharges from hospital in the last year of people's lives.

The views of relatives and others

Fifteen per cent of respondents for people who had died at home felt at some stage that it would have been better for the person to be in a hospital, hospice or other institution. The proportion who felt they would have been better at home when they died in hospital or other institution was similar: 11 per cent.

Respondents were more critical about the stage of admission and discharge. Twenty three per cent of those who could answer the question felt that admission to hospital had been too late, less than one per cent that it had been too soon. When the person who died had been discharged from hospital during the last year of their lives and subsequently readmitted to the same hospital 13 per cent of respondents felt they should have been kept in and not discharged. Another ten per cent made some other comment about this, so almost one in four had some reservations about the discharge. Most of their comments related to the inadequacy of services and support outside the hospital.

Conclusion

These observations of the extent and distribution of the care given by the hospital service to people in the last year of their lives raise a number of issues. One is whether, given that the care of people who will be dead within a year is so large a part of hospital work, hospitals are adequately equipped and staff adequately trained in the skills needed for this type of care. The traditional orientation of the hospital towards diagnosis and cure may not be geared to meet people's needs for symptom relief and supportive care. As Williams (1990) puts it:

> Medical students are likely to be over impressed by the capacity of modern medicine to cure, as throughout their course they will be heavily exposed to pharmacological and surgical approaches.

Chapter eight showed that there was better pain control in hospices and that respondents were generally more satisfied with the care that had been given in hospices. Yet, as argued in the last chapter, hospice care is almost entirely devoted to cancer patients and people dying from cancer tend to be younger, are more often married and less likely to live alone than people dying from other causes. Hospice services are focused on their needs, but the needs of chronically ill, older people who are less likely to have near relatives to care for them seem less likely to be met by either hospice or hospital services. These are the people who are most likely to be in residential or nursing homes (the subject of the chapter that follows), and the observation that they are relatively unlikely to be admitted to, or to die in, hospital suggests that a careful evaluation of their possible needs for hospital or hospice care should be made. It may be that they are avoiding unnecessary investigation, over treatment and the stress and potential disorientation of change. But it could be that they are being denied helpful therapy and skilled and specialised care from which they would benefit. Fentiman et al. (1990) have argued that cancer in the elderly is often badly treated and this may be so for other conditions too. A survey of general practitioners (Pell et al. 1990) found that most would opt for hospital care for patients with uncomplicated myocardial infarction who were under 70 but would treat older patients at home, depriving them of the benefits of thrombolysis.

The pattern of shorter stays and more frequent admissions of patients to hospital in recent years is another cause for concern for people in the last 12 months of their lives. These may be acceptable and indeed preferred if there is adequate support and care in the community. But when this is not available hospitals may be seen as a relative haven. The appropriate balance of care between hospital and community is another issue to be resolved, and will be discussed in Part IV.

11 Residential and nursing homes

The marked rise in the number of residential homes, particularly the recent growth in the private sector (DHSS 1987, Bebbington and Tong 1986, Laing 1985) has drawn attention to the somewhat uncertain role of these homes (Judge and Sinclair 1986). Two areas of concern are: first, who should have residential care and second, the relationship between residential and community care. In this chapter we look at the characteristics of the people who spent some or all of the last year of their lives in residential and nursing homes and at the care they got from general practitioners, community nurses and hospitals. Care and conditions in the homes and the extent of visiting are described and a final section considers the quality of people's lives as perceived by their relatives and others.

Types of home and numbers receiving care

The "homes" covered in this study include residential homes for older people, nursing homes and other institutions excluding hospitals or hospices. For convenience they are referred to here as residential homes. Fourteen per cent of the sample of deaths occurred in such homes; this compares with a much lower proportion, 5 per cent in 1969 (Cartwright, Hockey and Anderson 1973).

A further 9 per cent of the people who died spent at least part of the last 12 months of their lives in such homes; so almost a quarter, 23 per cent, were in residential homes at some stage in the last year of their lives. The length of time they spent there and the types of homes involved are shown in Table 11.1. Those classed as other homes included convalescent homes, a rehabilitation centre, an assessment centre, a holiday home for the disabled and rest homes which may in practice have been homes for older people (the classification was made on the basis of the information given by the person interviewed). A relatively high proportion of those in other types of home were there for less than a month. Sixty two per cent of those in old people's homes had been there for a year or more compared with 47 per cent of those in nursing homes, but this difference might have occurred by chance.

Of the old people's homes, 56 per cent were said to be run by the Council, 6 per cent by a charity and 39 per cent were private.[1] In contrast the great majority of nursing homes, 83 per cent, were privately run. Nearly a quarter of those in nursing homes had not had to pay towards the cost of living there compared with only 7 per cent of those in old people's homes. The reason for the difference seemed to be that the DHSS paid for nursing home treatment in a number of instances. As one person said: "They took the pension and attendance allowance and the DHSS paid the rest."

Nevertheless the proportion for whom payment was thought to have been something of a problem was 7 per cent of all those in old people's homes (15 per cent for private ones, 6 per cent for others) and 17 per cent of those in nursing homes (further differences which did not reach statistical significance).

Table 11.1
Length of time spent in different types of home

	Old people's homes	Nursing homes	Other homes	All residential homes
	%	%	%	%
Less than a month	10	17	(44)	16
1 month < 3 months	10	12	(6)	10
3 < 6 months	5	5	(6)	5
6 months < 1 year	13	19	(13)	15
1 year < 2 years	23	20	(6)	20
2 < 5 years	25	22	(19)	24
5 < 10 years	10	5	(6)	8
10 years or more	4	-	-	2
Number of residents (=100%)	87	41	16	145*

Percentages in brackets are based on less than 20 cases.

*Includes one for whom the type of home was not known and excludes two for whom the length of stay was not known.

Who spent time in a residential home?

Age, sex and family

People who lived longer were more likely to have spent some or all of the last year of their lives in residential homes. People have been counted as spending all of the last year of their lives in residential homes if they had lived in one for a year or more. In fact, as will be seen later, a number of them were admitted to hospital during the last 12 months of their lives and some died in hospital. Few under 75 had spent any time in such homes but more than half those dying when they were aged 85 or more had spent at least some of the last year of their lives in one. The figures are in Table 11.2 which also shows expected age related differences with sex and marital status.

Table 11.2
Characteristics of people spending some or all of last year of their lives in residential homes

	Proportion spending		Number of deaths (=100%)
	some time	all last year	
Age at time of death			
Under 65	4%	2%	142
65 - 74	8%	1%	147
75 - 84	24%	10%	203
85+	56%	37%	147
Sex			
Men	12%	5%	301
Women	33%	19%	338
Marital status			
Single	33%	21%	81
Married	7%	2%	288
Widowed etc.	38%	21%	263
Any living brothers or sisters			
Yes	15%	8%	383
No	35%	19%	217
All deaths	23%	12%	639

Further analyses by age and marital status showed that married people less often spent any time in residential homes than single or previously married people of the same age. The proportions among those aged 75-84 were 8 per ent of the married, 34 per cent of the others, and for those aged 85 or more 25 per cent compared with 61 per cent. Neill et al. (1988) found that few married people applied for residential care and those who did so were less likely to be admitted than applicants who were single or widowed. There were no significant differences on the present study between the never and the previously married although it might be expected that people with children might be less likely to go into a home than those without any and the widowed, divorced or separated were much more likely to have children than the single: 75 per cent compared with 6 per cent. An analysis by marital status and number of children showed that for the married the main difference was between those with no children, 17 per cent of whom had been in a residential home, and those with one or more, for whom the proportion was 5 per cent. For the widowed or divorced there was no difference between those with and without children nor any significant trend with the number of children.

So it would seem that children may assist one parent to care for the other who might otherwise go into a home, but apart from this they have no effect overall. It may be that they encourage and facilitate admission to residential homes for some while caring for and thus avoiding the admission of others, and that these two influences cancel each other out in the statistics.

An analysis by the sex of children showed no significant differences between those with a son or sons only and those with only a daughter or daughters. The 1969 study found that those with a daughter or daughters were more likely to die in their own homes than those with just a son or sons.

Data in Table 11.2 suggest that those with living brothers or sisters may be less likely to be admitted to a home. Part of this is an age effect: the proportion with such relatives falling from 86 per cent of those aged 45-54 to 41 per cent of those aged 85 or more. Among those aged 85 or more a similar proportion of those with and without living siblings had been admitted to a home at some stage but among those aged 75-84 more of those without any such relatives had been admitted: 30 per cent compared with 17 per cent. These variations reflect the fact that siblings themselves age and die and therefore become less of a source of support as people grow older.

Cause of death

People who died of cancer were less likely than those dying from other causes to have been in such homes 7 per cent compared with 29 per cent.

The difference remains when the age at which they die is taken into account. When the type of home was taken into account, those dying of respiratory disease were more likely to have been in nursing homes (14 per cent compared with 6 per cent for those dying of other conditions) whereas those dying of stroke were more likely to have been in old people's homes: 27 per cent compared with 12 per cent.

Self care

The proportions reported to have had difficulty with various aspects of caring for themselves (see p.82) for a year or more before death was 87 per cent of those who had been in a residential home for a year or more, 60 per cent of those in for a shorter time and 25 per cent of those who had not been in such a home at all. (People who had been in a hospital for all the year before they died have been excluded from these comparisons). But many of the symptoms asked about were reported for similar proportions of those who had been in residential homes and those who had not; these were pain, trouble with breathing, vomiting or feeling sick, drowsiness, sleeplessness, dry mouth or thirst, depression, loss of appetite, difficulty swallowing, dizziness, bed sores, an unpleasant smell and backache. However, for a number of these symptoms, more people in residential homes had had them for a year or more: the proportions were 31 per cent compared with 20 per cent for drowsiness, 22 per cent compared with 14 per cent for dizziness, 19 per cent compared with 11 per cent for loss of appetite and 4 per cent compared with one per cent for bedsores. Only one symptom, a persistent cough, was reported more often for those who had *not* been in a residential home (24 per cent compared with 10 per cent of those who had spent some time in such a home). When deaths from cancer were excluded the difference remained: 22 per cent compared with 9 per cent.

Symptoms

The symptoms reported more frequently for those in residential homes are shown in Table 11.3. Several of them - constipation, confusion, urinary incontinence and difficulty seeing and hearing - have been shown elsewhere to increase with age (Cartwright 1990). Some of them, such as mental confusion, incontinence and difficulty seeing and hearing, may have contributed to them being admitted to such homes. They can certainly make it more difficult for people to look after themselves. Among those people with confusion, constipation and incontinence, those in residential homes were more likely to have had the symptoms for a year or more. The figures were 81 per cent compared with 39 per cent for confusion, 78 per cent and

52 per cent for constipation and 54 per cent compared with 36 per cent for incontinence.

Bad temper might result from being in such a home. Another explanation for the relatively high proportion of those in residential homes reported to be bad tempered could be that relatives, friends or neighbours were less likely to report or perceive the person who died as being bad tempered than staff of institutions. Among those in residential homes the frequency with which bad temper was reported was 31 per cent when the respondent was a relative, friend or neighbour, 45 per cent when he or she was a staff member (a difference which did not reach statistical significance). But if the comparison between those who had been in a home and others is confined to those for whom relatives, neighbours or friends were interviewed, there is still a difference: 31 per cent compared with 19 per cent. Bad temper could be either a cause or effect of being admitted to a residential home. Other studies have found that caring relatives are more likely to favour residential care as a solution for the elderly confused if the old person exhibits difficult behaviour (Levin et al. 1989).

So the evidence suggests that because of their age and frailty those living in residential homes will have needed more care during the last year of their lives than other people who died.

Table 11.3
Symptoms reported more often for people in residential homes

Symptom:	Person in residential home at some stage in last year of life	
	Yes	No
Mental confusion	59%	30%
Constipation	45%	34%
Dribbling	21%	11%
Bad temper	35%	19%
Loss of bladder control	58%	26%
Loss of bowel control	36%	19%
Difficulty seeing	34%	21%
Difficulty hearing	46%	23%
Number of people who died (=100%)	147	492

Care from general practitioners

People in residential homes remain under the care of general practitioners. The numbers of consultations, home visits and night calls reported for those in such homes for a year or more before they died are compared with those for others under the care of a general practitioner in Table 11.4.

Table 11.4
Consultations, home visits and night calls in the last 12 months of their lives for those living in residential homes and others under the care of general practitioners

	Those in residential homes all year	Others	All under care of general practitioners
All consultations	%	%	%
0	-	6	5
1-4	18	32	31
5-9	31	21	22
10-19	30	22	23
20+	21	19	19
Home visits			
0	-	23	20
1-4	20	38	36
5-9	31	15	17
10-19	29	13	15
20+	20	11	12
Night calls (8pm-8am)			
0	75	73	73
1	16	12	12
2-4	7	11	11
5-9	2	2	2
10-19	-	1	1
20+	-	1	1
Number of deaths excluding those in hospital all year*	78	545	625[a]

* The 14 who were in hospital for all the 12 months have been excluded altogether.
[a] Includes two for whom the length of time in a home was not known.

As expected, those in residential homes had more consultations and more visits from their general practitioners than others. But, if anything, they had rather fewer night calls. Of course night calls are usually made in a crisis and the help normally available in residential homes may make it easier to cope with a minor one without calling out a doctor.

In the minority of homes (a quarter) where all the residents had the same doctor, visiting rates were higher (16.8 a year on average) than in the majority (three quarters) where the residents could have different doctors (9.5). However the proportions for whom the general practitioner was described as reluctant to visit, or for whom it was felt it would have been helpful if the doctor had visited the person who died more often, did not vary significantly between the groups. So it would seem that people in homes where they were free to have a doctor of their own choice were not seen as being more deprived of visits in spite of having fewer of them than people in homes where everyone had the same doctor. Those in homes where everyone had the same doctor might receive less individual attention at visits if general practitioners saw several patients on the same visit.

The mixture of praise and criticism for general practitioners' care of people in residential homes was similar to comments about their care of others during the last year of their lives. Although most respondents praised, or were satisfied with, this care the study identified a number of inadequacies. Home visits were much appreciated when they happened but failure to visit was one of the more common and significant criticisms.

> The matron of a residential home, talking about a doctor who she felt was reluctant to visit and said it would have been helpful if the person who died had been visited more often: "It would have given her a lot more comfort and the staff a lot more confidence." When asked why she thought the doctor had not come more often, she replied, "The doctors feel the residents are in a rest home to save them working." The doctor had not been asked to come more often "because we're resigned to the fact that, unless it's an emergency, he won't come out." The matron also told us that this person had to go into a nursing home "towards the end" because "she needed morphine injections which the doctor wouldn't give otherwise she wouldn't have had to move to somewhere strange. She had to leave her room, her furniture: that's why she gave up."

Care in hospital

People who had lived in old people's homes were less likely than others who died to have gone into a hospital or hospice during the last year of their lives or to die in one. This can be seen from the figures in Table 11.5 which also suggest that the longer the time they had lived in an old people's home the less likely they were to go into hospital. But those least likely to have spent time in a hospital or hospice or to die in one were those who had lived in a nursing home for a year or more.

Table 11.5
Variations in proportion admitted to hospital in the last year of their lives with stay in residential homes

	Proportion who died in hospital or hospice	Proportion in hospital or hospice at some time in last year	Number of deaths (=100%)
Not in residential home at all	59%	81%	492
In old people's home less than a year	48%	76%	33
1 year < 2 years	} 39%	65%	20
2 years or more	}	53%	34
In nursing home			
Less than a year	45%	91%	22
1 year or more	0%	16%	19

This lower use of hospital in-patient facilities was not accounted for by the older age of the people in residential homes although fewer of all those aged 85 or more had spent time in hospital (64 per cent compared with 80 per cent of those under 85). Among this older group 46 per cent of those who had been in a residential home for a year or more were admitted, 75 per cent of the others. There were similar differences when people dying of respiratory disease and of cerebrovascular accident were considered separately: the proportions admitted to hospital were 25 per cent and 47 per cent of those in a residential home for a year or more, 76 per cent and 89 per cent of others among the two cause of death groups respectively. The numbers dying of other causes were too small to analyse separately.

The only source of information from this study of any possible reluctance to admit people from residential homes to hospital relates to those who were admitted and respondents' views on whether they should have been admitted earlier. This showed that in practice relatively few, one in ten, of those who had spent any time in residential homes were thought to have been admitted to hospital "too late"; this proportion was a quarter for those who had not spent any time in a residential home.

Residential homes, and long stay nursing homes in particular, appear to cut down the use of hospital care during the last year of people's lives. What of the nursing care given by district and other nurses to those in old people's homes?

Help from visiting nurses

Just over a third, 35 per cent, of those who had lived in an old people's home for a year or more had had help from a nurse who visited the home in the year before they died. This was similar to the proportion receiving help from district and other nurses among those who had not spent any time in such homes once sudden deaths and those who had spent all their last year in hospital have been excluded. They also received similar numbers of visits.

Given their age, symptoms and frailty, it might have been thought that the residents of old people's homes would receive more care from visiting nurses than people in the community, as they received more visits from general practitioners. But some of the less skilled tasks undertaken by district and other nurses for people living in their own homes were probably done by staff in the residential homes. The next section looks at respondents' views of the care given to people in residential and nursing homes and the conditions there.

Care and conditions in the homes

Almost nine tenths, 88 per cent, of the people who had spent some time in a residential home were said to have had access to a telephone where they could make calls and people could telephone them. Among those who did not have this facility, two fifths were thought to have wanted it. Ninety two per cent of those in old people's homes compared with 82 per cent of those in other sorts of homes had this amenity (a difference which fell short of statistical significance) but more of those in old people's homes had a room of their own, two thirds compared with half. Overall the proportion with a room of their own was three fifths and again two fifths of those without one were thought to have wanted one.

If the respondent was a relative, friend or neighbour, they were asked to say whether they thought various aspects of the home were good or not so good. The replies of those who felt able to make these assessments are shown in Table 11.6. Clearly their views may have been different from those of the people who died, but respondents are likely to have taken into account the reactions of their relatives and friends, and how these respondents felt about the care in the homes is also of interest and concern.

Table 11.6
Views of relatives, friends or neighbours on various aspects of the home

	Food	Heating	Deceased's room	Bathroom & lavatory facilities	Stairs or lift	Other things about building	Way home was run
	%	%	%	%	%	%	%
Good	71	91	81	93	74	92	80
Not so good	16	6	14	6	12	5	14
Other comment	13	3	5	1	14	3	6
No. of respondents (=100%)	79	85	84	81	77	74	79

The most frequent criticism was of the food, and over this there was a difference between old people's homes for which 26 per cent thought the food "not so good" and nursing homes for which it was 7 per cent. There were no differences between Council homes and private ones on any of these assessments, nor in the amenities available. The overall assessments of the homes were similar in the two groups and between nursing homes and old people's homes. Altogether 50 per cent were described as "excellent", 31 per cent as "good", 9 per cent as "fair", 6 per cent as "poor" and one per cent as "dreadful", with 3 per cent making other comments.

A number of criticisms were exacerbated by feelings that people were in the wrong type of institution. A son whose father had Parkinson's disease and had been in an old people's home commented:

> They were not equipped to deal with a progressive condition, they were not that kind of establishment. The degree of mental stimulation was absent. It was a very distressing time for him. The whole point of his

being there was because of his condition. He could have been in a hotel, had he not needed care and supervision which he blatantly did not get.

The daughter of a woman with Huntingdon's chorea who had been in a nursing home described the care she got there as: "Limited - not because they didn't want to care, they just didn't know how to care for this type of patient... It should not be registered as a nursing home."

The one "dreadful" home was thought to have contributed to the death of the man admitted there:

> It was an awful place: dreary, badly furnished and he wasn't as clean as he'd been in hospital - food all down his clothes and he hadn't shaved, he really looked unkempt. I don't think the staff cared. I'm sure the fact of moving to the home contributed to his death. He was so well when he left hospital... and the deterioration within a week was unbelievable. I just feel he gave up when he got in that home. (Died of Parkinson's disease and pneumonia aged 73 within 24 hours of being readmitted to hospital after being in an old people's home for less than a month).

A number of respondents commented on the lack of stimulation. As one put it: "They sat in the front room and didn't move. Just sat there, no TV and no one seemed to talk to them."

When asked about the other residents in the homes, respondents' views were roughly equally divided about whether the person who died had on balance found them helpful (25 per cent) or tiresome (22 per cent). Most of them, however, 53 per cent, made other comments, generally to the effect that the person had had little to do with other residents: "Her mind had gone so she was not able to socialise."

Many of the relatives and friends who rated the homes as an excellent place for the person who died to live towards the end of his or her life made rather perfunctory comments: "I can't fault the home," "It was very nice, no qualms about it." Others were rather more forthcoming:

> I would say that, instead of "spoon feeding" the residents, they tried to make them independent. The staff were always there to help but didn't impose themselves. This was very good and they kept her there when they could have sent her to hospital. (Friend of woman who had had a number of strokes).

A wife whose husband had had multiple sclerosis and went to a holiday home for the disabled for two weeks to give her a rest said:

It's a good idea, gets them away from home to meet new people. They deserve a holiday like everybody else. He had a good time, said he really enjoyed it and would like to go again, and I had all the washing done for me. He didn't bring anything home dirty except the previous day's clothes.

Sometimes relatives and the people who died had obviously had different views of the home. One daughter-in-law who rated the home as excellent went on to explain that her mother-in-law:

hated everything about everything. We thought they were angels in the home and that everything was marvellous. The staff told us she was the most difficult lady; as far as she was concerned nothing was right. She had to share (the bathroom and lavatory) much to her annoyance, but they were just next to her room. You get what you pay for.

The views of people who had previously looked after those who died sometimes reflected their gratitude and admiration for the people who took on this task. A friend of 30 years standing who had previously cared for a woman with senile dementia described how:

I thought she was just being awkward until she slowly went downhill and became incontinent. I got help from the social services for this: they brought sheets and pillowcases from the hospital. The crux came when she became doubly incontinent and her mind had got to the point where she had forgotten how her body functioned. It was winter and I was changing her clothes three times a day and my self control snapped and I shook her very hard to stop her sitting down without her pants and was so upset by my behaviour and frightened by what I had done that they agreed to put her in a home. The young nurses were very kind and would kiss and cuddle her.

Visiting

How much contact do people in residential homes have with relatives, friends and neighbours outside? This question is considered for people who had been in such homes for a year or more. The number of different visitors they were reported to have had during the last 12 months averaged 5.0. Seven per cent had none, 52 per cent had one to four, 33 per cent five to nine, and 8 per cent ten or more. The number of visits was much greater: 11 per cent had 300 or more (almost one a day), 33 per cent between 100 and 300 (two or more a week on average), 19 per cent 50-99 (between one and two a week), 4 per cent 20-49 (between one a fortnight and one a week), 14 per cent 10-19 (less than one a fortnight), 12 per cent had less than 10 (less than one a month). The number of visits was strongly related to the number of visitors: of those with less than five visitors, a quarter had a hundred or more visits, but this proportion was three quarters for those with five or more visitors. Of those who were visited, 44 per cent had only relatives to see them, 11 per cent were visited just by friends or neighbours and 45 per cent by both relatives and friends; the most frequent visitor was a relative for 78 per cent and a friend or neighbour for 22 per cent.

Three of the five who had no visitors were said by the people we interviewed to have had no relatives. Neither of the other two who had no visitors had any children; one had elderly relatives abroad, the other, in the opinion of the deputy officer in charge of the home, only had herself to thank: "Because of her awkward manipulative ways she just didn't get any visitors. She did get visits from other visitors but they wore off because of her awkwardness... She went out of her way to be unpleasant to people."

Isaacs et al. (1972) found that relatives' failure to provide basic care for elderly people was often associated with their previous rejection by the elderly person. However, for one in five of the people in residential homes for a year or more, our respondents said that there were relatives who they felt might have visited more often. This compares with one in four of those living in the community who were felt to have relatives who might have helped more (a difference which might well occur by chance).

Quality of life

Respondents were asked whether they would describe the quality of life of the person in the year before they died as good, fair or poor. Two things appeared to affect this assessment independently. One was whether the respondent was a staff member or a relative. Those spending any time in a residential home were less often described as having a poor quality of life if the respondent was a staff member than if he or she was a relative: 10 per cent compared with 42 per cent. This probably reflects the perceptions of the respondents rather than a real difference in the actual quality of life of the people who died, although staff members may have been more willing to act as respondents for residents they had got on well with, and those residents may have had a better quality of life because of their relationship with the staff.

The other factor that was related to assessments of quality of life was whether people had been in a residential home for a year or more or for a shorter time. Taking all types of respondents together their ratings were similar for people who had not been in a residential home at all and those who had been in one for a year or more, while those who had only spent part of the last year of their lives in a residential home were generally felt to have had a worse quality of life: for 39 per cent of them it was rated as poor compared with 27 per cent of the other two groups. The difference between those spending all and those spending some of the last 12 months in a home persisted when the analysis is confined to those for whom relatives responded. This can be seen in Table 11.7. In addition, among those for whom a staff member responded only one in 12 of those admitted during the last year of the life was felt to have had had a good quality of life during that time compared with nearly half (46 per cent) of those who had been in a home for a year or more.

Table 11.7
Quality of life analyzed by time in residential home for those for whom relative responded

Quality of life in last year	Time in home		
	Not in residential home at all	Admitted in last year	In home all year
	%	%	%
Good	36	13	35
Fair	28	37	24
Poor	28	46	38
Other comment	8	4	3
Number of deaths for whom relative responded (= 100%)	346	48	34

One possible explanation for these findings is that people take time to adjust to living in residential homes. Another possibility is that those going into residential homes shortly before their death do so in a crisis situation. Weaver et al. (1985) found that residents most able to come to terms with admission were those who had exercised some degree of control or choice in entering residential care. Findings from the present study suggest that once people had become established in the homes their quality of life, in the opinion of their relatives, was similar to that of other people who died and had never been in such homes.

Conclusion

Most of the people, just over two thirds, who spent all the last year of their life in a residential or nursing home were 85 or more, and it is this age group which is predicted to increase most rapidly in the next 20 years (CSO 1989) so it is likely that increasing numbers will spend the last year of their lives in such homes. But this increase may not be as great as the rise in the numbers of older people if there is an improvement in their state of fitness as Jefferys and Thane (1989) suggest.

The symptoms that were more common among those in residential homes, particularly confusion, incontinence and bad temper, indicate some of the problems in making these homes attractive and stimulating places to live. The description of one man of 94 illustrates many of the difficulties:

> He wasn't ill, it was just general deterioration. He was still quite active for his age, but his mental deterioration was the problem, he'd lost his sense of direction. He found it difficult to accept his own failings. Memory loss was the worst aspect, the fact that he was unable to complete a crossword puzzle in ten minutes as he once could troubled him. He was suffering from frustration. He was worried because he was deaf, worried because of his bowels. He worried a lot. He was, I think, unhappy and tired. He often said he'd had enough of living and was "ready to go" was how he put it. (Died from falling down a flight of steps and fracturing his skull).

That man was admitted to hospital after his fall and died there within a week without regaining consciousness. But in general people living in residential homes were less likely than others either to die in, or to be admitted to, hospital during the last year of their lives. Residential homes seem to cut down the use of hospital care, they probably also reduce the need for it, but this is less certain. They may also reduce the demand and need for night calls from general practitioners and, taking into account the age and frailty of residents, the pressures on the district nursing service.

Because of the nature of the sample this study could not ascertain the views of residents themselves. Others who have done so have argued that elderly people are often faced with a choice between an unpleasant battle to survive in their own homes and an equally unpleasant enforced dependence in the institution (Wilkin and Hughes, 1987). In this study relatives and friends generally thought conditions in the home were "good" rather than "not so good", although a number of their comments and descriptions indicate that circumstances were sometimes far from ideal and analysis of respondents' views of the quality of life suggest that the initial period after admission may be particularly stressful for residents. While most residents were in fairly frequent contact with relatives and friends from outside the home, one in five of those who spent all the last 12 months of their lives in a home had either no visitors at all or less than one visit a month. Becoming old and frail can be distressing; to be also isolated from relatives and friends seems dire.

The task of relieving avoidable distress and creating a caring and heartening environment in residential and nursing homes is going to be of increasing importance in determining the quality of the last year of people's lives.

Notes

1. A few of the people in the sample may have been in the same home. The homes were not identified so it is not possible to be certain.

12 Day centres[1]

Two of the key objectives of the government proposals for care in the community are: "to promote the development of domiciliary, day and respite services to enable people to live in their own homes wherever feasible and sensible," and "to ensure that service providers make practical support for carers a high priority." (Secretaries of State for Health, Social Security, Wales and Scotland 1989).

One branch of day care services consists of day centres, and their intended aims coincide with the above objectives: helping people to remain independent in the community and providing support and relief for those relatives, friends and neighbours who are carers. Day centres aim to give social care, stimulation and company for those attending as well as a number of personal care services, such as provision of meals, bathing facilities and chiropody as well as other treatment such as occupational therapy, physiotherapy and medical care (Brocklehurst and Tucker 1980, Tester 1989, Tuffnel and Warburton 1981). Attenders do not usually initiate contact but are referred by general practitioners, social workers, wardens of sheltered housing schemes and from hospital (Fennel 1979).

Other authors have noted the distinction between day centres and day hospitals (Donaldson et al. 1987, Tester 1989, Wadsworth et al. 1972), the main emphasis of day centres' being social care and the maintenance of independence in the community, while day hospitals place greater emphasis on treatment and rehabilitation for people after discharge from hospital or to prevent in-patient admission. However, in practice, the distinction is not clear, and referral can be more dependent upon availability of day care services than on theoretical objectives.

In this chapter no distinction is made between day centres and day hospitals, but respondents were asked who the day centres were run by. By comparing and contrasting the experiences and care of those who attended day centres with those who did not, and by looking at those for whom respondents said such attendance would have been helpful, the role day centres do and could play in the last year of people's lives is examined.

People who attended day centres

Numbers attending

According to respondents' reports, 57 (9 per cent) of the people who died had attended a day centre at some time during the final year of their lives. Of these, 58 per cent attended a centre run by social services, 34 per cent one run by a hospital, 6 per cent one run by a voluntary organization, and one person who died had attended a private day centre.

Over half, 55 per cent, had been attending for a year or more before they died, 20 per cent between three months and a year and a quarter less than three months. Twenty two per cent attended four or more times a week, 71 per cent two or three times a week, and 7 per cent once a week or less often. The average number of times a week people had attended was just under three.

Those using centres run by hospitals attended for shorter periods of time than those using centres run by others (only 33 per cent of those using day centres run by hospitals had attended for a year or more, compared with 65 per cent of the others). This could be a reflection of one of the aims of day hospitals, the rapid rehabilitation of people discharged from hospital in-patient stays (Wadsworth et al. 1972).

Demographic characteristics

As can be seen from Table 12.1, those who lived longer were more likely to have attended a day centre at some stage during the last 12 months of their lives. Only 5 per cent of those who died under the age of 75 attended a day centre compared with 13 per cent of those aged 75 or over. As will be clear by now, age is a key variable as it is associated with a number of other characteristics including declining activity (Qureshi and Walker 1989) and increasing symptom prevalence (Cartwright 1990).

The fact that the majority (63 per cent) of attenders were women is a reflection of the greater age of attenders, as women live longer than men. Another age related variation is the difference in proportions of attenders and non attenders who were widowed, a difference which disappeared when age at death was taken into account. However, age did not account for the differences in household composition also shown in Table 12.1. Of those aged 75 and over at death, 50 per cent of attenders compared with 32 per cent non attenders lived alone, still a significant difference.

Cause of death also revealed differences which could not be explained by the age variation. People who had attended a day centre in the final year of their lives were less likely to have died of cancer (7 per cent of attenders died of cancer compared with 29 per cent of non-attenders). Conversely, those who had attended a day centre were more likely to have died of a stroke (35 per cent of attenders compared with 11 per cent of non attenders died of a stroke) and of mental disorders (11 per cent of attenders compared with two per cent of non attenders). When these analyses were restricted to

Table 12.1
Age, sex, marital status and household composition by day centre attendance in the last year of life

	Non attender	Attender	All
Age:	%	%	%
15-44	4	-	4
45-64	19	12	18
65-74	25	14	23
75-84	30	49	32
85+	22	25	23
Women	51%	63%	53%
Marital status:	%	%	%
Single	13	14	13
Married	48	36	46
Widowed	36	50	38
Separated	3	-	3
Lived:	%	%	%
Alone	26	40	26
With others	61	48	58
In hospital/residential home all year	13	12	16
Number of deaths (=100%)	547	57	639*

*In 35 cases it was unknown if the person who died had attended a day centre. In 21 of these the person who died had lived in an institution for the whole of the last year of their lives.

those aged 75 and over at death, the differences remained: 5 per cent attenders compared with 19 per cent of non attenders died of cancer; 38 per cent of attenders compared with 16 per cent of non-attenders died of stroke, and 12 per cent compared with 3 per cent died of mental disorders.

Those who had attended day centres in the last year of their lives, then, had different characteristics to non attenders and some of these characteristics (living alone and dying from conditions other than cancer) were not simply reflections of the greater age of attenders. It was shown in chapter five that people living alone were least likely to have living children or siblings and were most likely to be widowed or divorced, and in chapter nine it was shown that deaths from causes other than cancer were associated with long term symptoms and restrictions. Thus, those who attended day centres appear to have been a frail group of people with fewer potential sources of care from family members, a group of people with greater need of formal care services, including day centres.

Table 12.2
Experience of long term restriction[a] by day centre attendance in the last year of life

	All ages Attended			75 and over Attended		
	No	Yes	All	No	Yes	All
Needed help to:	%	%	%	%	%	%
Get in/out of bath/shower	26*	60	31	41*	62	46
Dress/undress	13*	40	16	19*	36	22
Go to toilet	9*	25	11	13	21	15
Wash (and shave)	9*	26	11	14*	26	16
Feed himself/herself	4*	14	4	5*	17	6
Cut own toenails	36*	77	41	55*	84	60
Make hot drink	16*	41	20	25	34	28
Help at night	12*	35	15	19	26	21
Any other thing	12*	26	14	18	24	20
At least one of the above (except help with toenails)	32*	67	36	47*	67	51
Number of deaths (=100%)	533	57	625	270	42	339

*Difference between attenders and non attenders significant at the 0.05 level or beyond.
[a]Experienced for a year or more before died or went into hospital/hospice for the last time. Those who were in hospital all year are excluded.

Symptoms and restrictions

Respondents' reports reveal that the people who had attended a day centre at some stage in the final year of their lives were more likely than the others to have had long term difficulty with all the restrictions of daily living asked about (that is they had had difficulty caring for themselves for a year or more before death). When the analyses were carried out excluding those

Table 12.3
Experience of long term symptoms[a] by attendance at a day centre in the last year of life

	Non attender %	Attender %	All %
Pain	40	46	41
Trouble with breathing	28	20	27
Vomiting/feeling sick	10	14	11
Drowsiness	22*	33	23
Sleeplessness	23*	38	25
Dry mouth/thirst	15	22	16
Mental confusion	16*	46	20
Depression	20*	39	22
Loss of appetite	13	19	13
Difficulty swallowing	7	9	7
Constipation	19*	31	21
Persistent cough	16	11	15
Dizziness	15*	31	16
Dribbling	4*	14	5
Bad temper	14	18	15
Bed sores	2	4	2
Incontinence	12*	27	14
Unpleasant smell	5*	14	5
Difficulty seeing (with spectacles)	17	21	18
Difficulty hearing	23	32	25
Backache	22	29	22
Other	17*	28	18
Total number of deaths (=100%)	547	57	639

*Difference between attenders and non attenders significant at 0.05 level.
[a]Experienced for a year or more before death.

aged under 75 most of the differences remained significant. The results are shown in Table 12.2.

Respondents were also asked whether the person who died had suffered from a number of symptoms and for how long the symptoms were experienced. The comparisons between attenders and non attenders are shown in Table 12.3. Several of these symptoms have been shown elsewhere (Cartwright 1990) to increase with age. However, when the analyses were restricted to those aged 75 and over, two symptoms were still significantly more likely to be experienced by attenders on a long term basis. Those who had attended a day centre in their final year were more likely than those who had not to have suffered from long term mental confusion (45 per cent compared with 25 per cent), and sleeplessness (45 per cent compared with 27 per cent).

These differences in the prevalence of symptoms and restrictions confirms the picture of those who had attended day centres as particularly frail. Among the more elderly, attenders were still more likely to have required long term help with bathing, dressing, washing, feeding and toe nail cutting, and they were more likely to have suffered from long term mental confusion and sleeplessness. This indicates that those who attended day centres were a group particularly in need of support. It also gives an indication of the high demands placed on family and friends caring for this group of people. All these factors probably contributed to the initial need for day centre care.

Day centre care

According to respondents' reports, the day centre arranged transport to and from the centre for 82 per cent of those who had attended. However, nearly a quarter (23 per cent) of these attenders were said to have experienced problems, usually related to the tardiness or cancellation of the transport. One respondent, the wife of a man who died of a pulmonary haemorrhage, aged 70, commented:"They forgot to tell him they weren't going in bad weather; he stood outside and got pleurisy." Another, the daughter of a 69 year old woman who died of cerebro-vascular disease, said: "She became confused if she waited for the ambulance too long; she became confused on the journey, she thought she was being taken away from home." It is clear from such comments that transport is an area of great concern.

Respondents were also asked how the person who had died had spent their time at the day centre, and this is shown in Table 12.4. Thus, most people participated in some form of social activity at the centre. Of the respondents who mentioned "something else", ten specified recreational activities such as bingo, films or outings, five hairdressing, four chiropody, two mentioned discussion groups giving welfare advice, and one said the person who had

Table 12.4
What did he/she do at the day centre?

	%
Chatted to other patients	87
Had lunch	84
Chatted to staff	81
Had occupational therapy	43
Did handicrafts	38
Had exercises/physiotherapy	32
Had a bath or shower	24
Something else	52
Number of attenders (= 100%)	57

died had had speech therapy at the centre.

Those who attended a day centre run by a hospital were more likely to have had exercises or physiotherapy there than those who had attended centres run by others: 69 per cent compared with 14 per cent. This is again indicative of the differing emphasis of day hospitals: on ambulatory and medical care, with a view to rehabilitation, enabling the patient to continue with activities of daily living (Donaldson et al. 1987). There were no other significant differences between those using centres run by hospitals and those run by others in the activities reported.

Respondents were asked how much attenders enjoyed their days at the centre. Just over half, 53 per cent, of people who had attended a day centre in the final year of their lives were said by respondents to have enjoyed their days there a lot, 25 per cent some or a little, and 17 per cent were said not to have enjoyed their days at the centre at all (other comments were made by the rest).

Those who lived alone were more likely to have enjoyed their days at the centre (74 per cent enjoyed their days there a lot compared with only 37 per cent of those who lived with others). What attenders did at the day centre seemed to have some effect on how much they enjoyed their days there. Only 35 per cent of those who had exercises or physiotherapy at the centre were said to have enjoyed their days there a lot compared with 67 per cent of those who did not take part in these activities. Of those said *not* to have chatted to other people at the centre, two fifths did not enjoy their days there at all compared with only one tenth of those who did chat with other people.

Reasons for not enjoying the visits ranged from indifference: "She was indifferent to the visits, so wouldn't mind if she went or not" (Son of a woman who died of stroke having suffered from senile dementia for many years), to outright loathing: "Absolutely hated it. He hated the bother of going in the ambulance and waiting about; he didn't like the people who went - they played bingo which wasn't his style" (Friend of a 73 year old man who died of bronchopneumonia).

Respondents were also asked how helpful the visits to the day centre were to them or others who had looked after the person who died. Fifty seven per cent said they were very helpful, 7 per cent fairly helpful, 11 per cent said they were not helpful, and 25 per cent made other comments. Of those who said they were very helpful 11 made specific comments, and of these eight indicated that the visits gave them a break from the demands of caring. Two of the respondents who said attendance at a day centre by the person who died had not been helpful made specific comments. The husband of a 52 year old woman who died of pneumonia following an overdose of aspirin said, "The staff didn't seem to care. They said "go for walks" in the pouring rain." A son whose 88 year old father died of a heart attack said, "I used to worry all the time he was away and wonder if he was alright, so that really it didn't give me any rest at all."

Sometimes the interests of the carer and the cared for seemed to be in conflict. The wife of a man who died of a heart attack, aged 65, having survived a stroke seven years earlier reported that the visits to the day centre had been very helpful to *her*, but commented, "I used to say "it's for your own good" but if he'd had his way he wouldn't have gone at all. In those last years he just wanted to be here (at home) and I'd get nothing done at all." Another, the daughter of an 85 year old woman who died of a stroke, again reported that the visits had been very helpful to her, but said:

> She went one week and liked it. Second week she said she wasn't going. Third week she absconded. She went into the house opposite (the day centre) and told them to "get out of my house." She fought the staff when they went to get her... But just fancy, an old woman, your own mother of 85, absconding!

Care at home from nurses and home helps

Were those who attended day centres more or less likely to have received domiciliary care? Just over half, 51 per cent, of those who had attended a day centre had been visited at home by a nurse in the year before they died. Surprisingly, given the pattern of symptoms and restrictions, this was similar to the proportion of those who did not attend who received help from a nurse at home.[2] The frequency of visits and the period of time over which visits were received were also similar. Nor were there any differences between the groups in the proportions said to be in need of some nursing care (if they had not received any) or of more nursing care (if they had). It may be, given the nature of the symptoms and restrictions that were more prevalent among day centre attenders, that practical support and assistance was needed more than nursing care.

This would appear to be confirmed by the observation that home helps seem to have played a greater role in supporting those who attended day centres. Fifty per cent of attenders had had a home help in the last 12 months of their lives compared with only 22 per cent of those who did not attend a day centre in their final year.[2] Even so, 34 per cent of those who had attended a centre were said to have been in need of such help or of more help, compared with only 22 per cent of non attenders. Among those aged 75 and over at death attenders were still more likely to have had a home help than non attenders: 56 per cent compared with 35 per cent (though there was no difference in the proportions thought to be in need of such help or of more help).

It is probable that those who attended day centres were more likely to have received home help for the same reasons as they went to the day centre: they are a group of frail, elderly people living alone with few sources of informal care, needing assistance from formal care services to remain independent.

Care in hospitals and residential homes

One of the aims of day centres is to help people to live in their own homes wherever feasible. However, 63 per cent of attenders had spent a month or longer in an institution (hospital and/or residential or nursing home) in the year before they died compared with only 43 per cent of those who had not attended a day centre. But this was a reflection of the age variation between the two groups. When the analyses were restricted to those aged 75 and over at death, the difference disappeared. Given the prevalence of long term symptoms and restrictions among attenders, it seems likely that day centres do help to prevent people with high levels of need and frailty from spending time in institutions.

Those for whom attendance at a day centre may have been helpful

Respondents reporting on people who had not attended a day centre in the last year of their lives were asked if it would have been helpful if they had been able to go. Of those who answered this question, 49 said it would have been helpful, 11 per cent of the total sample of deaths for whom this information on attendance was available.[2]

Thirty four respondents who said attendance would have been helpful made specific comments, mainly related to why the person who died had not attended a centre. Four respondents mentioned that the person who died had been too ill to attend a day centre, two said that there were problems with transport, and two said that care at a day centre had not been offered. However, the majority, nearly three-quarters of all those who commented, said that the person who had died had not wanted to go to a day centre, "He didn't want to go, he didn't want anyone but me to look after him" (Wife of an 83 year old man who died of cancer of the bladder). Sometimes, this unwillingness seemed to have been resented by the respondent, "She was bloody stubborn, she wouldn't go. She had the opportunity. It would have been a break for me, especially when it was bad weather and she wouldn't go out" (Son-in-law of an 84 year old woman who died of pneumonia). Of course, for those for whom respondents said it would have been helpful but for whom specific comments were not made, there may have been other reasons for not attending, including, for example, lack of knowledge of available services.

Eighteen respondents gave reasons why attendance at a day centre would have been helpful. The most frequently given reason (by nine respondents) was that it would have provided respondents with a break from the demands of caring. One respondent, a daughter whose 85 year old mother died of cardio-respiratory failure, said, "The doctor arranged it but... when the bus came she flatly refused to go. It would have been nice for me to have one day a week to myself, perhaps to go out to lunch." Five respondents mentioned that attending a day centre would have provided the person who died with friendship/company, two said it would have been "a change", and the rest made other comments.

Characteristics

Were the needs and attributes of those for whom respondents said day centre attendance would have been helpful any different from those who had attended a day centre in the last year of their lives? The demographic attributes of the two groups were very similar: analysis by sex, age, marital status and who the person who died had lived with in their last year of life revealed no significant differences.

The only difference between the two groups in the experience of long term symptoms and restrictions was that those for whom respondents said attendance would have been helpful were more likely to have suffered from a persistent cough for a year or more before death (27 per cent compared with 11 per cent). This is a reflection of the finding that those for whom respondents said attendance would have been helpful were more likely to die of respiratory disease than those who attended (18 per cent compared with 5 per cent). They were less likely to die of a stroke (12 per cent compared with 35 per cent of attenders).

Given the similar characteristics of the two groups, it is useful to examine possible differences in the receipt of other care services. Were those for whom respondents said attendance at a day centre would have been helpful more likely to be receiving assistance from nurses or home helps or were they more likely to spend time in institutions?

Care from nurses and home helps

Similar proportions (just over a half) of those for whom respondents said attendance at a day centre would have been helpful and of those who had attended, had been visited at home by a nurse in the year before they died. But of those who had not been visited by a nurse, 59 per cent of the former group were said to have needed nursing care compared with only 9 per cent of those who had attended a day centre.

Furthermore, those who attended a day centre were more likely to have received some help from a home help (50 per cent of attenders received such help compared with 28 per cent of those for whom respondents said attendance would have been helpful). Of those not receiving home help, 61 per cent of the latter group compared with only 24 per cent of attenders were said to be in need of such help. Of those who had home helps, there was no difference between the two groups in the proportions thought to have been in need of more help.

There seems to be a high level of need for more formal care among those for whom respondents said attendance would have been helpful. It could be that some of those people reluctant to attend day centres were also reluctant to receive help or care in the home from strangers and wanted to retain as much independence as possible. Lewis and Meredith (1989) in a study of women caring for their elderly mothers found failure to co-operate in care was a frequent occurrence: most common was refusal by the mother to consider the possibility of anyone else caring other than the daughter. Alternatively, lack of knowledge of available services could be a factor. Those already "in the system" and receiving some formal help and care may be referred to other services or they may have greater awareness of and therefore greater access to available services.

Institutional care

As one of the fundamental aims of day centres is to help people remain independent in the community it might be expected that those who attended a day centre would be likely to have spent less time in hospitals or residential homes in the last year of their lives than those for whom respondents reported that attendance at a day centre would have been helpful, given the similar pattern of symptoms and restrictions and demographic characteristics of the two groups. However, this did not appear to be the case. Considering the total time spent in an institution during the last 12 months of life, there were no differences between the two groups. Nor were there any differences when the amount of time spent in hospital only was considered. When the amount of time spent in residential or nursing homes only was considered, those who attended day centres were more likely to have spent six months or longer in such homes in the final year of their lives (19 per cent compared with 4 per cent), but this could be because residential homes may refer people to day centres.

Conclusion

The government is committed to an agenda for care in the community, including the promotion and development of day care services. Just under one in ten people identified from a random sample of deaths from all causes were said to have attended a day centre at some stage in the final year of their lives, according to respondents who knew them. Most of these centres were run by social services departments.

Those who attended day centres appear to be a sub group of elderly people, with a high level of frailty and fewer family sources of support and assistance available. This group of people were also more likely to have received home help in the last 12 months of their lives, but a greater proportion than non attenders were still said to be in need of such or of more help.

Most people who attended day centres took part in social activities such as chatting with staff and other people and fewer received personal care services such as bathing and chiropody at the centre. There was some indication of the different emphasis of day hospitals, on treatment and short term rehabilitation. The majority of people were said to have enjoyed the visits to the day centre, and most respondents said it had been helpful to them or others who had looked after the person who had died, mainly because it provided relief from the demands of caring. But on occasion there seemed to be conflict between the wishes of the carer and those of the cared for.

According to respondents it would have been helpful if a further 11 per cent of those who died had attended a day centre in the last year of their lives. In terms of demographic characteristics, symptoms and restrictions, those who had attended a day centre were similar to those for whom respondents said attendance would have been helpful. The most often stated reason why attendance would have been helpful was that it would have given the carer a break from the demands of caring, and the most often given reason why the person who died had not attended a day centre was that they had not wanted to. This group of non attenders appeared to be in greater need than attenders of a range of domiciliary and day care services, including community nursing and home help, according to respondents' reports. It could be those people reluctant to attend day centres were reluctant to accept care from strangers in their own homes. No doubt lack of access and knowledge of available services also plays a part. Those already in the formal care system may have greater access to all care services, creating a group of high users of services and a group of low users of services, though both with similar levels of frailty. The government apparently recognises that most care is provided by family and friends. Levin et al. (1983) reporting on a study of those caring for elderly mentally infirm relatives or neighbours cite the importance of community services in reducing stress in supporting relatives, and in chapter thirteen it is suggested that the absence of such services may make some relatives reluctant to take on the role of carer as this may mean taking on more responsibility than can be regarded as reasonable. Day centres play a significant role supporting those elderly people living alone with few sources of informal care and may help reduce stress in caring relationships by providing informal carers with a break. However, elderly people have usually been living independently most of their lives, and dependency and care may be difficult to accept, especially from people outside the family (Lewis and Meredith 1989, Qureshi and Walker 1989). A range of domiciliary and day care services suitable for the individual needs of both the cared for and their family and friends are necessary. Services available currently do not appear to be enough, are not always appropriate and do not always reach those in need.

Notes

1. This chapter was contributed by Graham Farrow who assisted us in the latter stages of the study.

2. Sudden deaths of people aged under 65 and those who spent all their last year in a hospital or nursing home have been excluded from these analyses, as respondents for these were not asked questions about home nursing.

Part III
CARE IN THE COMMUNITY

Introduction

As was shown in the last chapter day centres can play an important part in providing respite care, enabling those who might otherwise enter longer term institutional care to remain at home. It has long been government policy to encourage community care in this sense, and the adequacy of arrangements for care in the community were an important focus for the first study of *Life before Death*. Achieving the right balance between community and institutional care remains as important an issue now as it was in 1969. The 1969 study reported many general practitioners saying that there was a shortage of beds for elderly people needing long term nursing care, and concluded that this meant increased reliance on domiciliary services. These, particularly district nursing and home helps, were overstretched in 1969, with nurses reporting that they had inadequate time to spend in supporting patients and their relatives as they hurried from one house to another, and many respondents saying that the home help service was inadequate to meet the needs of the people who died.

The 1969 study also emphasised the need for better communication between the various services involved. In particular, difficulties were identified in the quality of communication between hospitals and general practitioners at discharge, and district nurses sometimes felt that an earlier referral and more information about patients at the time of referral from general practitioners would be helpful.

One aim of the 1987 study was to see if any of these things had changed during the period concerned, and the chapters in this part of the book address this issue. In addition, the influence of the changes that have occurred in general practice, community nursing and other community services since 1969 on the experience of care in the last year of life is assessed. It will be recalled from the introductory chapter that some of the most important changes were, as far as general practitioners are concerned, a growth in group practices, a decline in overall list size but a worsening ratio of general practitioners per head of the 75+ population (Table 1.3). There has also been a decline in home visiting by general practitioners (Table 1.4).

As for the district nursing service, it was shown that by 1987 there were fewer nurses per head of the 65+ population, although the number of people treated per nurse had risen, suggesting a more thinly stretched service (Table 1.5). Other domiciliary services, such as meals on wheels, home help and chiropody, have all increased in quantitative terms (Table 1.6). None of these trends distinguish services received by people in their last year of life. The chapters in Part IV help to identify the impact of such trends on this group.

In chapter thirteen the views of general practitioners, hospital consultants and community nurses about whether the right balance between hospital and community care was being achieved, is reported. In addition, the views of relatives, friends and others is drawn upon to judge this. The chapter looks again at some of the issues raised by the 1969 study: whether there are still difficulties in arranging long term nursing care and the perceived adequacy of coverage of the various community services. In addition, the chapter considers in some detail the adequacy of pain control at home. New approaches to pain control have been promoted by hospice practitioners (Twycross 1978) and it is an area in which specialist domiciliary terminal care teams claim expertise. Inadequate pain control in the home can be a significant factor in admission to a hospital or hospice, and thus affects the balance of care in the last year of life.

There follow two chapters in which two of the key community services are considered in depth: general practitioners (chapter fourteen) and community nurses (chapter fifteen). The decline in home visiting by general practitioners shown in national statistics suggest that those suffering from disabling illness preventing mobility, as many in our sample were, might be particularly hard hit by this change. Chapter fourteen pays particular attention to this issue, as well as exploring the role of training and qualifications in influencing the quality of service provided by general practitioners.

The adequacy of coverage of the community nursing service is of particular concern given the trends reported in chapter one. Chapter fifteen reports the perceptions of both nurses and relatives, friends and other respondents concerning the adequacy of this service. Given the concern expressed by some nurses in 1969 about late referral and inadequate information at referral from general practitioners, this issue is explored in detail in this chapter. In addition, pain control at home from the nurses' point of view is considered, since this has sometimes been an area of contention between nurses specialising in terminal care and general practitioners (Simms 1984).

The final chapter in this part of the book is about the relationships between the general practitioners, hospital consultants and community nurses involved in the study. Here, the issues of communication at discharge from hospital, the timing of referral to nurses by general practitioners, and views about the quality and need for specialist domiciliary terminal care services, are examined.

13 The balance of care

The balance of care between hospitals and the community is one of the major concerns in the health service. It has been recognised as an issue in the care of the dying for some time. Taylor (1983) argued that for the terminally ill, the development of home care services should take priority over further in-patient units. Parkes (1985) questioned this on the grounds that, while pain control for people with cancer had improved in the seventies, severe pain was still common among those who remained at home. As was shown in chapters two and ten, while the proportion of people dying in hospitals increased between 1969 and 1987, they had more frequent admissions and shorter stays in the more recent year. The views and experiences of three professional groups involved in the care of the dying, general practitioners, hospital consultants and community nurses, on the balance of care between hospitals and the community were sought on the 1987 study. Their opinions and observations are reported in this chapter, together with some information from relatives and others associated with the people who died. The issues considered are the appropriateness of the present balance of care, the adequacy of community care and of hospital and hospice services, and pain relief in hospital and at home.

The balance of care

All three groups of professionals were asked whether in their area they would like to see more care for the dying given at home, if people could be cared for there adequately, more in a hospital or hospice, or whether they felt the balance was about right. Replies are shown in Table 13.1. A majority of both hospital consultants and community nurses would like to see more care being given in people's homes if adequate care could be arranged

Table 13.1
Views on balance of care for the dying*

	GPs	Hospital consultants	Community nurses
Would like to see	%	%	%
More at home	43	57	59
More in hospital or hospice	8	10	5
Balance about right	49	27	33
Other comment	-	5	3
Don't know	-	1	-
Number (=100%)	239	204	92

*Excludes 6 general practitioners (2 per cent) and 7 hospital consultants (3 per cent) who did not answer this question.

Table 13.2
Views on further facilities needed in their area*

	GPs	Hospital consultants	Community nurses
	%	%	%
Short term general hospital beds	42	50	67
Chronic hospital beds	66	40	67
Geriatric beds	54	38	73
Mental hospital places	43	20	38
District nurse services	47	54	77
Home help services	63	63	87
None of these	3	5	-
Number (=100%)	245	198	86

*Excludes 13 hospital consultants (6 per cent) and 6 community nurses (7 per cent) who did not answer this question.

there. General practitioners were more evenly divided between those holding that view and those who felt the present balance was about right.

A list of various hospital and community resources was presented to the three professional groups and they were asked whether they thought more of each of the services were needed in their area (Table 13.2). Home help services were frequently mentioned by all three groups. General practitioners attached about the same importance to increasing chronic hospital beds. An increase in district nurses services was thought desirable by three quarters of the community nurses and by approximately half of the other two groups.

In response to another question, 8 per cent of consultants said they frequently had to keep patients in hospital longer than they otherwise would because of the inadequacies of the district nursing service, 42 per cent said they did so occasionally, 47 per cent rarely or never (the rest made other comments). A similar question about the home help service suggested inadequacies in that service caused rather more problems: 15 per cent of the hospital consultants said they frequently had to keep people in hospital longer, 46 per cent did so occasionally, 35 per cent rarely or never (the remaining 4 per cent made other comments).

Adequacy of community care

The nurses' views on the need for more help services were reinforced by their answers about the adequacy of the home help services in their areas: 36 per cent of them compared with 16 per cent of the general practitioners described them as "very inadequate." Hospital consultants were also asked this question, but a fifth of them said they did not know; among those who did answer the question replies were similar to those of the general practitioners.

All three groups were asked about a number of domiciliary services that might or might not be available in their area and whether they would like to see them introduced or extended (Table 13.3). One in eight of the consultants said they did not know whether the first three services were available in their area and a further 5 per cent did not answer the question; just over a quarter did not indicate whether they would like these services extended or introduced.

In addition to the substantial number of consultants who indicated that they did not know whether a service was available it would seem that others may have mistakenly believed that a night sitting or night nursing service was not available. More community nurses than general practitioners reported that the various services were available in their areas, except for a day care service for the terminally ill. The nurses were also more likely to want services extended or introduced, especially night sitting services, day care services for the terminally ill and night nursing services.

This desire of the nurses for an increase in night services ties in with their views on the changes they would like to see in the district nursing service or in the way it was organised. Over half of them (55 per cent) wanted to see some changes, compared with two fifths of the general practitioners and a third of the consultants. The most common change the nurses wanted was for more staff, and this was often related to their desire to spend more time with patients: "If there were more staff we could spend more time with patients and sit and chat if they don't have a caring family and friends."

The next most frequently mentioned change the nurses wanted was 24 hour cover for patients: "The problem is that we are essentially a visiting service and can't provide 24 hour care. We can go three times a day but that's not 24 hour care. We need some kind of bank of nurses who, if necessary, could be with the patients 24 hours, and Marie Curie sitters seven nights a week instead of two."

Table 13.3
Availability of community services and views on whether they should be introduced or extended

	Available			Want extended or introduced		
	GPs	Consultants	Nurses	GPs	Consultants	Nurses
Night sitting service	74%	51%	90%	41%	49%	66%
Night nursing service	70%	47%	89%	38%	51%	53%
Day care services for terminally ill	39%	41%	36%	40%	47%	60%
Geriatric social worker	36%	70%	63%	37%	22%	44%
Number (=100%)*	240	183	92	240	157	91

* Totals exclude people who did not answer the question, or who did not know whether the service was available.

When relatives were asked for their views, one in five felt that it would have been helpful if the general practitioner had visited the person at home either at all or more often. They thought that one in eight of those who had not had any help at home from a district or other type of nurse could have done with some help from a nurse during the year before they died, and just over a fifth, 22 per cent, of those who had had help from a nurse were thought to have needed it more often.

For one third of the people who had died and who had been living alone, relatives thought there should have been more help with shopping, cleaning or cooking. The proportion was similar for the 79 people who had had a home help from the social services (50 per cent of those who lived alone) and those who had not. Among the 365 people living with others, only 14 per cent had had a home help, and 37 per cent of those with such help were thought to have needed more help with the shopping, cleaning or cooking, compared with only 15 per cent who had not had a home help. So it would seem that those who were living alone were seen as less likely to get such help if they needed it, and that the help they got was felt to be inadequate for one in three of those living alone and for a similar proportion of those living with others.

Adequacy of hospital and hospice services

General practitioners, hospital consultants and community nurses were all asked about the availability of hospice beds. Three quarters of both groups of doctors and two thirds of the nurses said there were some in their areas. The proportions wanting this service introduced or extended were 35 per cent of general practitioners, 46 per cent of hospital doctors and 58 per cent of community nurses. General practitioners were asked whether they found it easy, rather difficult or very difficult to get admission into a suitable NHS institution for a variety of patients. Admission was thought to be the easiest in the case of an elderly patient with an acute infection (86 per cent of respondents), but a few (3 per cent) said this was very difficult. The admission of a young patient with a short term terminal illness was described as easy to obtain by 81 per cent of general practitioners, with two per cent reporting it as very difficult, whereas an admission of an elderly person with a short term illness was seen as easy by 73 per cent of respondents and very difficult by 6 per cent. The people who were most often found to be difficult to arrange admission for were an elderly patient needing long term nursing care (17 per cent easy, 29 per cent very difficult) and a young patient with a progressive degenerative condition (18 per cent easy, 28 per cent very difficult).

Relatives and others were asked whether they felt people who had been admitted to hospital during the last year of life had been admitted too soon or too late, and for those who had been discharged, whether this had been done too soon. Nearly a quarter of people (23 per cent), were thought to have been admitted too late and less than one per cent too soon. Eleven per cent were thought to have been discharged too soon or inappropriately.

The issue of possible over treatment in hospital was raised in a question to general practitioners. Seven per cent thought over treatment of patients who were terminally ill happened very often, 33 per cent fairly often, 55 per cent occasionally, 4 per cent never (1 per cent made another comment). Some comments related to why or how over treatment occurred: "But how can young doctors be expected to take such decisions? Consultants are often not involved." Some related to the nature of the over treatment: "Useless attempts at chemotherapy make patients more ill." Others concerned the characteristics of patients who were over treated: "Over treated patients tend to be younger." A few doctors remarked that under treatment in hospital was more common than over treatment for patients who were terminally ill.

Relatives were asked whether there was any treatment the person who died should have been given in hospital but was not. They thought this had happened in 8 per cent of hospital episodes, a hospital episode being one or more admission to the same hospital during the last year of a person's life. One view on what should have been done and why it was not came from a daughter whose mother aged 76 died of cancer of the bladder: "They should have kept closer tabs on her diabetes. They're so busy with other things, old people don't matter much."

A similar proportion of relatives (6 per cent), thought that the person who died had been given some unnecessary treatment or operation during a hospital episode and a further 11 per cent were uncertain about this. A daughter whose mother had died of cancer of the bladder said: "Blood transfusions made her a bit better but prolonged the agony." A son who said his mother had died of old age, bed sores and pneumonia said: "With hindsight, a skin graft (for leg ulcer). She had to keep still and developed another bed sore. The sister on the ward said the decision to do the skin graft was bad medicine - inadequate communication between consultant and nursing staff."

Pain control at home and in hospital

Consultants and general practitioners held similar views about the proportion of dying patients for whom pain could be controlled satisfactorily (Table 13.4).

Community nurses were asked a rather similar question about patients dying at home and about the proportion of patients whose pain was satisfactorily controlled. Like the doctors, most of the nurses (87 per cent) thought it was possible to control pain satisfactorily for 80 per cent or more of patients dying at home. But over a third of them thought it was controlled in a smaller proportion than it could be. A number described the problems of determining the appropriate drug and dose and arranging help when needed. Some ascribed the discrepancy to the reluctance of patients to take drugs. Others were critical of general practitioners or felt there was a more widespread lack of knowledge: "A lot of GPs tend to stick to dosages they know, and they are reluctant to increase them. It's not like being in hospital with consultants always available." Inadequate liaison was also blamed and a few mentioned more than one cause: "Sometimes a patient denies pain and says he's pain free and sometimes GPs are not aware of pain and not giving enough analgesics."

Relatives and others who answered questions about people's lives in the year before death may have been more aware of any shortcomings in the care provided at home than of what happened in hospital. Certainly more of the relatives were unable to answer a question about pain relief in hospital than pain relief at home (17 per cent compared with 11 per cent). But the observations and opinions of those who were able to answer the questions suggest that pain was more likely to be treated in hospital than at home (96 per cent compared with 91 per cent) and that the hospital treatment was

Table 13.4
Doctors' views about proportion of instances in which pain in dying patients can be satisfactorily controlled*

	Consultants	General practitioners
	%	%
All	14	9
80% < 100%	72	72
60% < 80%	12	15
40% < 60%	1	3
20% < 40%	-	1
Less than 20%	-	-
Other comment	1	-
Number (=100%)	203	235

*Excludes 8 consultants (4 per cent) and 10 general practitioners (4 per cent) who did not answer this question.

more effective. Nineteen per cent thought that when pain was treated in hospital it was relieved completely all the time, whereas the corresponding proportion for pain treated at home was 9 per cent, and the proportions saying the treatment did not relieve the pain at all was 3 per cent for hospital care, 10 per cent for care at home.

Conclusion

The response rates from two of the three professional groups surveyed were only 62 per cent and 65 per cent respectively for general practitioners and consultants. Those who were less interested in care of the dying may have been less likely to participate. Another point of concern is that so many of the consultants, between one in eight and one in five, said they did not know about the availability of various community services in their area, and as many as one in four did not answer questions about whether or not they would like these services introduced or extended. Indeed the lack of knowledge, and apparent apathy, of some consultants about community care can be seen as an important finding of this study as it is likely to affect attempts to change the balance of care between hospital and community.

Few, 10 per cent or less, of each of the three professional groups wanted to see more care for the dying given in hospitals or hospices. In contrast, between two and three fifths would have liked to see more of this care given in people's homes, if it could be done adequately. But it is clear from their replies to other questions and from the views and experiences of the relatives of people who died that more resources are needed in the community if this is to be achieved. In particular more home helps, more district nurses and more night nursing and night sitting services are called for. In addition, as is shown in chapter fourteen, one in five relatives felt that it would have been helpful if the general practitioner had visited the person at home either at all or more often.

Community nurses reported that pain was not controlled satisfactorily for patients dying at home as often as it could be, and there was some evidence from relatives that pain control was better in hospital than at home. Some people may be willing to accept rather more pain, or delays in pain relief, for the other comforts and advantages of remaining in their own home. That said, it is obviously important and desirable that distressing pain, particularly in people who are dying, should be relieved as effectively and quickly as possible. Findings about inadequate pain control at home are supported by the observation that rather more than half the general practitioners (54 per cent) indicated that it would be helpful to have more training in the management of pain. With the rapid developments in the techniques of pain control such further education is likely to be an ongoing need. This in turn demands the participation of consultants who are specialists in this field, and they need to be aware of services outside the hospital.

It may well be that the absence of adequate supporting services in the community makes some people reluctant to take on the task of caring for their relatives, realising that if they do they will have to take on more responsibility than could be regarded as reasonable. If that is so, the clear inadequacy of so many of the community services may jeopardize what has been up to now the most important source of care and support for people in the community during the last 12 months of their lives. That in turn will put further demands on the hospital service and lead to the balance of care being tipped in an unsatisfactory direction.

14 General practitioners

Most people are under the care of their general practitioner for a large part of the last year of their life. This chapter is about the care people get from their general practitioners during this period, the views and assessments by their relatives and others of the quality of this care and about the views of general practitioners on caring for people who are dying. It also looks at the way this care varies with the characteristics of the patient, the illness and the doctor.

Frequency and nature of consultations

The people in the sample generally had several contacts with their general practitioners during their last year of life. The estimated numbers are based on information from the people we interviewed. Some of these respondents, one in eight, felt unable to make any estimate and for others it may have been difficult for them to make accurate assessments. In addition, they may not have been aware of all the consultations that occurred. Excluding the few who spent all the year in hospital and those for whom no information was available, the estimated average was just under ten consultations and this rose to ten and a half if sudden deaths with no illness or warning or time for care were excluded. The distributions for all consultations and for home visits and night calls are shown in Table 14.1.

A relatively high proportion of the contacts, about two thirds, were home visits and roughly a tenth were night calls. Even so, one in five did not have any home visits during this time and the majority, nearly three quarters, had no night calls. Among people dying at home and those dying in hospital the number of consultations were similar but those dying in hospices (4 per cent of the sample) were more likely to have had 20 or more consultations with their general practitioners, 36 per cent compared with 19 per cent of those dying at home or in hospital. This reflects the greater contact that people dying of cancer had with their doctors, compared with those dying of other conditions (see chapter nine).

As was shown in chapter two, the number of home visits was less in 1969. On the earlier study 30 per cent of the people who died in their own home had less than five home visits, on this study that proportion had doubled. This reduction in home visiting has happened even though people were dying

Table 14.1

Contacts with general practitioners in the last year of life

	%
All consultations	%
0	5
1	3
2-4	28
5-9	22
10-19	23
20 or more	19
Estimated average	9.8
Home visits	%
0	20
1	9
2-4	27
5-9	17
10-19	15
20 or more	12
Estimated average	6.8
Night calls	%
0	73
1	12
2-4	11
5-9	2
10-19	1
20 or more	1
Estimated average	0.9
Number of people* (=100%)	625

*Those in hospital all year are excluded from the table.

Table 14.2
Variation in the number of home visits and night calls with age during the last year of life

Age at death	Estimated average no. of home visits	night calls	No. of deaths on which average based
Under 55	5.3	1.3	57
55-64	4.9	1.1	72
65-74	5.9	0.8	137
75-84	6.9	0.8	169
85 and over	9.5	0.6	119

at an older age on the more recent study and home visits increased with age. This age trend is shown in Table 14.2. There is a clear trend apart from those dying under 55, a relatively high proportion of whom died from cancer (37 per cent compared with 25 per cent of older people). In spite of their comparative youth those dying from cancer had an estimated average of 8.5 home visits compared with 6.1 for those dying of other causes. By contrast, those dying of ischaemic heart disease had a lower than average number of home visits: 5.2, but several of these deaths were sudden ones with no previous illness or time for care: 18 per cent compared with 5 per cent of deaths from other causes. People with cancer also had more night calls than other people: 1.4 compared with 0.6, but night calls seemed to decline with increasing age.

People who lived alone had fewer consultations than those who lived with others: 8.1 compared with 10.2. But the difference in the average total consultation rate between the single, 8.6, and the married or previously married (for both of which it was 10.0) did not reach statistical significance, although the RCGP/ OPCS/ DHSS (1990) study found that adults who were single consulted less frequently than those who were married, widowed or divorced. That study also found that people living in council housing were more likely to consult than those in owner occupied housing. This study found no differences between owner occupiers and council tenants (a possible index of social class) in the number or place of their consultations with general practitioners. The 1969 study also found no social class variations in the number of general practitioner consultations, home visits or night calls and concluded that "death in many respects appeared to be the equaliser it is so often reputed to be." More surprisingly, men and women did not differ significantly in the total number of consultations reported but women had more home visits than men: 8.0 compared with 5.5, a reflection of the older age of women at the time of their death.

Most, 73 per cent, of the people who died who consulted a general practitioner at all saw only one or two different general practitioners (including partners, locums or deputies) in the last 12 months of their lives; 25 per cent saw three or four and two per cent five or more. For those seeing more than one 16 per cent of the respondents felt it would have been better to have fewer doctors, and this proportion was 25 per cent if the person had seen more than two doctors. A son whose father had seen five or more doctors said: "When you have one doctor for one patient it must be better. They know the case better and can see if the person is improving or not. Each doctor has their own ideas and so they start to argue with one another about what to do. They all think different."

Respondents' views of general practitioners' care

Most of the people we interviewed who could answer our questions about the care the person who died got from their general practitioners[1] described that care positively: 87 per cent thought the doctor was an easy person to talk to, 82 per cent that he or she had time to discuss things, 83 per cent felt the way the doctor looked after the person who died was very (63 per cent) or fairly (20 per cent) understanding and 74 per cent described the care the person who died got from his or her general practitioners in the last year of life as excellent (41 per cent) or good (33 per cent). On the obverse side there were criticisms. One in ten thought the doctor was not an easy person to talk to.

> Not easy at all. More of the old school. You tell him what is wrong and he gives you something, but no explanation. Sort of "I know best." I think he probably thought we couldn't cope with knowing Dad was dying. But it was the very thing we needed to know. I think he's frightened of telling you how it is. When we were desperate and tried to get it from him he just wouldn't communicate. (Son).

Fourteen per cent thought the doctor did not have time to discuss things: "They always seem to be in such a tearing hurry" (Wife); "He explained at first, then seemed to tire of her. My mother found her illness (Parkinson's disease) difficult to accept and probably kept asking the same things" (Daughter).

Eight per cent felt the general practitioner was "not very understanding." A husband whose wife had died of cancer described the three doctors his wife had seen as easy to talk to and said they had time to discuss things but felt they were: "not caring, technicians rather than doctors. You get a tablet and that's that, they're not interested."

Seven per cent described the general practitioner's care of the person who died as "poor". The sister of a woman who died of heart failure described the care her sister got from her general practitioner as:

> Awful; the doctor neglected her. He did nothing, showed no interest. He wouldn't come to see her. Once she went to the surgery, early last year. It took her four hours to walk there and back, then she had to wait over one hour to see him at the surgery. He showed no understanding at all, no interest. All he did was write a prescription. He didn't examine her. She wasn't fit. When I sent for him he said he didn't do home visits and she should go to see him. I told him she wasn't well enough, that was when he wrote to her, telling her to go to see the specialist. She just wasn't well enough to go. When she was really ill at the end the home help sent for me. When I got there she was so ill I rang the doctor. He wouldn't come. Then the home help rang him. He still wouldn't come. Then we got hold of the supervisor from the home help service. She came and immediately rang the doctor. She said if he didn't come she would ring the police doctor. He finally came. When he saw her he couldn't get to the 'phone quick enough to 'phone for the ambulance. It was too late, of course. She died later (within a week) in hospital. I have complained to the Family Practitioner Committee but they wrote to say I had to make a formal complaint and go to see them. I am so upset about it and at my age I get so distressed I didn't feel I could go through with it. (Sister aged between 65 and 74).

That example includes complaints that were made by a number of people: failure to examine and writing prescriptions rather than doing things. It also highlights the most frequent criticism which was over home visiting. Fourteen per cent thought the doctors were rather reluctant to visit and 21 per cent felt it would have been helpful if the doctor had visited the person who died at home, either at all or more often. They made this last criticism more often when the person lived alone than when he or she was living with others (29 per cent compared with 19 per cent) and as stated earlier, people living alone had fewer home visits.

Respondents' summing up of the different aspects of care the people who died got from their general practitioner was strongly related to the number of home visits they had had: the proportion describing the care as fair or poor (rather than excellent or good) was 28 per cent for those who had had less than five home visits in the year before they died, 16 per cent for those with five to nine home visits and 5 per cent for those with ten or more.

When the doctor had visited 20 or more times few respondents, 8 per cent, thought he or she should have done so more often. This proportion rose with the declining number of home visits to 33 per cent for those who had between two and four visits, but fell again to 19 per cent for those with none or one, presumably because those people were, generally, felt by both doctors and relatives not to need such care.

For most of the people for whom it was felt that it would have been helpful if the doctor had visited at all or more often, the doctor had not been asked. But for 16 per cent this had happened, and the doctor had not come: "He felt he couldn't do any more for her. He once said he didn't like dealing with old people" (Daughter whose mother had Parkinson's disease).

> He said there was no point on a couple of occasions, he could not help her. He seemed to lose patience with her as she got worse. At first he thought it was Alzheimer's disease because she was quite rational at times. But as time went on she became more and more confused and he seemed to get annoyed because she got people to contact him. He didn't seem to realise just how it was affecting us. We didn't know sometimes if we were coming or going. She needed to be constantly watched. (Daughter).

One person was clearly difficult. His son-in-law told us that, "He'd assaulted the doctor and the doctor was very reluctant to see him. He would not let them look after him." A wife whose husband had had an operation for bladder trouble in the year before he died said:

> You felt that if at all possible you had to go to the surgery. The receptionist made it difficult when you called to ask them to come out. They asked lots of questions. In the end, couldn't be bothered, went to surgery. Then when he took bad one night with pains in the chest it took two and a half hours to get the doctor to call. He sent for the ambulance. He was taken to hospital and put on a machine in intensive care. But he died of a heart attack.

A daughter who said the doctors had come when asked and described her mother's doctors as willing to do home visits qualified this by saying, "They would come out when you asked them but they never followed the visits up." She felt it would have been helpful if they had visited her mother more often: "They would have seen the change in her, that she was getting worse... She had had sickness and diarrhoea for about four months. The doctor just gave her medicine and said she was O.K. They looked at her and said it was nothing nasty." (Died of cancer of the liver).

Another daughter who felt it would have been helpful if the general practitioner had visited her mother said he was not asked because her mother

> was satisfied to talk to the receptionist and did not push the doctors to call. She would call the doctor and speak to the receptionist who would ask her what was wrong and what she wanted and send a prescription. (She took paracetamol all the time) You don't seem to be able to get a doctor out of his surgery now, especially old people, they are not forceful enough to ask to see the doctor, they just accept what the receptionist says. My mother was always saying how thoughtful the receptionist was when she called, and always asked her how she was, but that didn't get the doctor out to see her... If my mother had been seen regularly then the deterioration might have been noticed.

Her mother only saw a general practitioner once in the year before she died and that was the emergency doctor whom her brother called and who admitted her to hospital where she died within three days of pulmonary oedema, acute left ventricular failure, macrocytic anaemia and myocardial degeneration, and acute lung abscess. The death was certified by the coroner after a post mortem.

While the most frequent criticism was about reluctance or failure to visit, some of the most bitter comments seemed to be related to what was seen as failure to diagnose a problem early enough. The mother of a young (35-44) woman who died of cancer told us that her daughter had complained of various pains for nine months but the doctor said nothing was wrong with her. The daughter consulted her general practitioner at least ten times in the year before she died and had one home visit. The mother described the way the doctor looked after her as:

> Neglect. He's an old man and kept telling her she looked too well to be ill. He gave her all sorts of pills for stomach and back pains. Then she collapsed at work and they took her to the hospital and the young doctor who saw her was horrified. They did all sorts of tests and found she was full of cancer. If it had been diagnosed at the beginning they might have saved her.

A wife whose husband died of Hodgkin's disease, aged 35-44, also felt it might have been cured if it had been caught early enough. As it was "the disease went into his spine and that left him paralysed. (Later he) lost bladder and bowel control, then finally his kidneys packed up and that was it." He also had rheumatoid arthritis. He'd had 100 or more visits from a nurse in the last 12 months of his life but saw the doctor "hardly at all," between two and four times. The wife described the care from his general practitioner as "bad, very, bad. He (the doctor) just never seemed interested, very abrupt. He's weird, even the district nurse thinks that. It always seems as if he's in a hurry; everything has to be quick. It's just the reaction you get from him. He's talking to you and going out of the door at the same time."

Even if these relatives were mistaken in thinking that earlier diagnosis and intervention would have prevented the death of their daughter or husband, it is clear that they did not get the support they wanted from the general practitioner while caring for their dying relative.

The last two illustrations might suggest that respondents were more likely to be critical of general practitioners over the care given to young people who died, but this was not so. Nor were there any notable differences with cause or place of death, or with our index of social class (housing tenure) except that for owner occupiers the doctor was more often regarded as not easy to talk to: 14 per cent compared with 7 per cent for council tenants. It may be that owner occupiers had high expectations but an alternative explanation is that doctors are less relaxed, or less approachable with people they perceive as nearer their own status. Apart from those already mentioned over visiting there were no other differences in respondents' assessments of the care given to those who lived alone and those living with others.

Praise was more common than criticism, and there were many descriptions of caring doctors and comments which indicate the things they appreciated about the way the doctor looked after the person who died. Visiting was clearly valued. "They came whenever we rang and said they would come any time, even if only for reassurance for mother" (Son). "When Tom wouldn't go to see him, I went and had a quiet word with him. Tom was so stubborn, he didn't like bothering the doctor, but he (doctor) said he would call just to see how he was. He did and it was a great help to us" (Wife). So were explanations and the time spent in giving these.

> He always takes time to explain and to be as helpful as he can be. He was so considerate at the time and since. Nothing is too much trouble for him. He told me what to expect and he was right. We couldn't have wished for better help and care. My husband had faith in him. (Wife whose husband died of cancer of the stomach).

> He's very easy to talk to. He is my type of doctor: straightforward. He takes time to explain what is wrong, how he is treating it, with what and why. He explained what was wrong with Harry. He said I must keep calm, try not to get too upset and to call him if I needed him. (Wife whose husband died of cancer).

People were grateful when doctors made arrangements for other types of care.

> To me he is like a brother. He talks sensibly and explains everything. When my mother started to be ill he said "You can't carry on like this." He got help during the day and I paid for help at night. Then he told me she was getting worse and really we must get her into a home. He said it was the best place for her. He arranged for the health visitor to come and take me to see the place. The care was 100 per cent, couldn't have been better. (Daughter whose mother had senile dementia and then a stroke).

Other favourable comments were: "She always said he was a good doctor and that she could talk to him. He sent her for the tests and things and came to see her regularly here" (Friend). "My husband didn't want to go into hospital for the hernia. The doctor was kind and persuaded him. He knew how upset he was about having to go into hospital again." Kindness and sympathy at the time of death were recalled with gratitude: "He put his arm round my shoulder. I said it still hurts, even though we were expecting it. He understood because he had lost a child himself not long before" (Son). Lack of feeling at this time was occasionally recalled, but
with resentment: "When my father died he saw father and said "Sorry Mrs... (mother), he's left us." That was all. I've never seen him since." This daughter said a locum came subsequently when she asked a doctor to come to see her mother. The locum was "a lady who let her talk and stroked her head and was sweet in herself."

A general practitioner was present at 5 per cent of the deaths that occurred at home and came to the home within an hour of another 61 per cent.

Although many more respondents made appreciative rather than critical comments about the general practitioner's care, sometimes the lack of criticism alongside the description of what happened seemed surprising. Thus, a daughter who described the care her mother had from the general practitioners as "reasonable" went on to say "If only he had taken more notice of her that Monday before she died he might have been able to do something for her. But he didn't give her a good examination. He just said she had wind and the pain in her chest was indigestion." Her mother died of congestive cardiac failure on the Thursday that week. Another daughter who described her mother's doctor as easy to talk to went on to say "You can always ask her things, it's just that she only gave half answers."

A wife whose husband had a stroke seven years before he died of a massive heart attack at home and who had needed help with nearly all aspects of personal care since his stroke had not been visited at all by a doctor in the year before he died. But she blamed herself: "If I'm honest he should have seen the doctor more often. My fault really." She'd taken him to the surgery between two and four times, but felt it would have been helpful if they'd visited him at home as "he used to get a bit worked up going to the surgery." But she hadn't asked them to come because she thought "it wasn't fair to trail them out. (The care he had was) good (but) I sometimes think if they'd taken his blood pressure more often... but they didn't."

Several informants commented on the unwillingness of the person who died to consult or "bother the doctor" or ask for a visit. A wife whose husband had "started with blackouts about three years before" he died, described the care he got from his general practitioners as excellent and said

> If we asked them they were always here straight away and did what they could. (But) they could not visit if he would not have them in. I would say many times let me call the doctor when he had his blackouts but he said "no, it will go away soon." He did not like doctors and did not like to bother them. (Died of cerebral infarction).

Another wife whose husband had been ill with schizophrenia for 15 years and who hanged himself said: "They did all they could. He did not like to see doctors often, he had enough of them when he was in hospital. (The general practitioner's care was) very good. There wasn't much they could do. He was beyond them." A husband related how

> I had always promised her I would not call the doctor unless she asked me to. We promised each other this years ago. At first she would not let me call him, but eventually she did. (The general practitioners' care was) very good. They, like me, just didn't realise how ill she was because she didn't complain and she was so strong willed she could cover up her pain and appear all right. The doctor came four times in ten days and the last time said she had to go into hospital. They took her in and did X rays and found she had lung cancer.

Some people seem reluctant to criticise doctors and others may not want to admit to themselves that their relative could have had better care in the time before he or she died. What did the general practitioners themselves feel about caring for people who were dying?

General practitioners' perspectives

Just over half, 56 per cent, the general practitioners who answered our questions felt that on the whole they were able to give enough time to patients who were dying, but 43 per cent felt they would like to give more time, with one per cent making other comments. Younger doctors, aged less than 45, were more likely to feel they would like to give more time to dying patients: 48 per cent compared with 34 per cent for older doctors. (This proportion was high, 64 per cent, among the 28 doctors who responded to the questionnaires but who could not be traced in the Department of Health files or whose name was not recorded there). More of the doctors who reported that they had been through a recognised vocational training scheme for general practice would like to have more time for this group of patients: 53 per cent compared with 35 per cent without such training. Of course, vocational training is strongly related to age: 20 per cent of those aged 45 or more had been on a recognised vocational training scheme, 70 per cent of the younger doctors. A three way analysis showed it was the younger doctors who had had a vocational training who differed from the others, 54 per cent of them wanted to spend more time with the dying, 34 per cent of the others, with no variation between the other three groups.

Doctors working in practices where the average list size was 2,500 or more (this information came from the Department of Health) more often felt they wanted to give more time to patients who were dying: 55 per cent compared with 36 per cent of those with smaller list sizes. Another characteristic which distinguished the two groups was wanting further training in different aspects of terminal care. The figures are in Table 14.3 and show that more than half the general practitioners wanted further training in three of the various aspects of terminal care asked about, and two thirds wanted further training in bereavement counselling. Haines and Booroff (1986) reported similar findings.

The question about wanting to spend more time with dying patients was not related to being a trainer or member or fellow of the Royal College of General Practitioners. It was similar for men and women doctors, for those who trained in Great Britain or Asia and did not vary with their practice involvement in vocational training or teaching of medical students. Possibly, given the relationships with wanting further training in terminal care, this question has identified doctors with a particular interest in, or concern for, people who are dying. If so, one might expect this to be reflected in the reports of our respondents about the care given to the people who died. But no differences emerged either in the views of the respondents about the care that was given or in the number of consultations and home visits reported for the people in the two groups.

Table 14.3
Proportion of general practitioners wanting more training in various aspects of terminal care by whether or not they would like to be able to give more time to patients who are dying

Proportion who would find it helpful to have further training in:	General practitioners who feel able to give enough time	General practitioners who would like to be able to give more time to patients who are dying	All
	%	%	%
Management of pain	48	64	54
Control of dyspnoea	51	64	56
Relief of nausea & vomiting	41	58	48
Communication with dying patients	50	66	56
Bereavement counselling	57	76	65
No. of doctors(=100%)	133	103	245

General practitioners were asked how easy or difficult they found it to cope with their own emotional reactions to death and dying. Just under two thirds said they found it easy (13 per cent) or fairly easy (52 per cent) and a third difficult (3 per cent) or rather difficult (30 per cent), with two per cent making other comments. (Nearly all this last group indicated that it was between fairly easy and rather difficult). They were also asked how easy or difficult they found it to cope with the emotional distress of terminally ill patients and their relatives. Rather more, almost half, found this difficult (5 per cent) or rather difficult (44 per cent). Responses to the two questions were strongly related: just over a third, 37 per cent, of those who found it easy or fairly easy to cope with their own emotions said they found it difficult or fairly difficult to deal with the distress of patients compared with almost three quarters, 74 per cent, of those who found it difficult or rather difficult to deal with their own reactions. Neither assessment varied significantly with the doctor's sex, country of qualification, whether he or she was a trainer or member of the Royal College of General Practitioners, nor was there any clear trend with the doctor's age in the doctor's ability to cope with their own reactions, but younger doctors reported more difficulty dealing with the emotions of patients or relatives: 57 per cent of those aged 45 or less said they found this difficult or rather difficult compared with 39 per cent of older doctors. Those with larger lists of 2,500 or more, were more likely to say they found it easy to cope with their own emotions: 23 per cent compared with 10 per cent of those with smaller lists. Fifty nine per cent of those with large lists compared with 46 per cent of those with smaller ones found it easy or fairly easy to deal with reactions of patients and relatives. There was no difference in the number of home visits made by doctors who found it easy or difficult to cope with either their own emotional reactions or those of their patients and relatives.

Respondents' assessments of the general practitioners' approachability and understanding were related to the doctors' assessments of their abilities to cope with their own emotions but not to their views on how easy or difficult they found it to cope with the distress of patients and relatives. More of the doctors who found it easy to cope with their own feelings were described as being easy to talk to: 97 per cent compared with 83 per cent of the others; and more of those who found it difficult or rather difficult to cope with their reactions were said not to have time to discuss things, 21 per cent compared with 11 per cent of those finding it easy or fairly easy. Fewer of those finding it at all difficult were described as having looked after the person who died in a way that was "very understanding" 57 per cent compared with 68 per cent of those who found it easier. It would seem as if the question about their own reactions has identified some doctors who have some problems in communicating with patients who are dying or with their relatives and do not respond to their needs so effectively. There was a clear trend in responses to this question and the doctors' wishes for more training over various aspects of care. This is shown in Table 14.4.

Doctors who said they had some difficulty coping with the emotional distress of terminally ill patients and their relatives were more likely than those who found it easy or fairly easy to want more training in communication with dying patients; 66 per cent compared with 47 per cent, and more training in bereavement counselling; 75 per cent compared with 55 per cent; but they were no more or less likely to want training in symptom relief.

But whether such training would improve doctors' ability to cope with their own or their patients' reactions is uncertain. There was no difference between those who said they had had some specific training in the care of the dying or management of bereavement and those who had not in their statements about their ability to cope with their own emotional reactions or with those of terminally ill patients and their relatives. And if such training was readily available it did not seem as if those in most need of it would be more likely

Table 14.4
Relationship between doctors' own emotional reactions to death and dying and views on further training

	Ability to cope with own emotional reactions to death and dying		
	Easy	Fairly easy	Rather difficult or difficult
Would find it helpful to have more training in:	Proportion thinking further training would be helpful		
	%	%	%
Management of pain	34	51	68
Control of dyspnoea	34	61	58
Relief of nausea and vomiting	28	47	57
Communication with dying patients	31	55	69
Bereavement counselling	34	66	77
Number of general practitioners (=100%)	30	125	79

to enrol for it than others; among those who thought it would be helpful to have more training in communication with dying patients the proportion who were described as being easy to talk to was 87 per cent compared with 82 per cent among those who did not think it would be helpful, a difference which might well occur by chance, but there were no differences significant or otherwise in the opposite direction. It may be that doctors with difficulty in coping with distress need help in understanding their own emotions rather than training in communication skills.

General practitioner characteristics and care

It might be expected that general practitioners who had had some specific training in the care of the dying or management of the bereaved would be more skilled or understanding in their care. A quarter of the general practitioners who answered our questions reported such training. This was more common among members or fellows of the Royal College of General

Practitioners 41 per cent of whom had such training compared with 21 per cent of non members, but there was no difference between those with such training in the views of respondents on the care given to the people who died nor in the number of consultations and home visits reported.

The frequency of home visiting did however appear to be related to the average list size of the general practitioner. The estimated numbers of home visits and other consultations are shown in Table 14.5; the main difference is for people with doctors in practices with an average list of less than 2000 (who had an estimated average of 8.0 home visits in the year before they died) and those whose doctors looked after 2000 or more patients (an average of 6.4 home visits). But our respondents did not regard doctors with larger lists as being more reluctant to visit nor were they more likely to say it would have been helpful if the doctor had visited the person who died more often. Those with larger lists may select their home visits more carefully and effectively than those with fewer patients to care for. There were no other significant differences in our respondents' assessments of the care given to the person who died with their doctor's list size.

The doctor's age was related to some of these assessments (see Table 14.6) with younger doctors coming out rather better in terms of being easy to talk to, having time to discuss things, being understanding in the way they looked after the person who died and giving them excellent care. This ties in with indications from other studies (Cartwright and Smith 1988, Bowling and Cartwright 1982) that elderly patients may have a more satisfactory relationship with younger than with older general practitioners. But unlike the other studies there was no evidence on this one of lower consultation or home visiting rates for people with older doctors.

Table 14.5
Estimated number of home visits and other consultations for patients of doctors with different list sizes

	Estimated number of consultations			Number of people who died(=100%)
	Home	Surgery	All	
Average list size				
Under 1,500	9.4	2.9	12.3	241
500-1,999	7.8	2.8	10.6	132
2,000-2,499	6.3	3.1	9.4	184
2,500 or more	6.6	3.2	9.8	106

Table 14.6
Variation with doctor's age in respondents' assessments of the doctor and his or her care*

	Under 35	35-39	40-44	45-49	50-54	55-59	60 or more
Doctor described as:	%	%	%	%	%	%	%
easy to talk to	98	92	76	76	88	84	91
not easy	2	5	22	22	10	12	7
other comment	-	3	2	2	2	4	2
Doctor thought to have:	%	%	%	%	%	%	%
time to discuss things	94	81	77	73	80	79	82
not	6	14	20	20	17	16	11
other comment	-	5	3	7	3	5	7
Respondent described the way the doctor looked after the person who died as:	%	%	%	%	%	%	%
very	71	70	55	60	61	68	64
fairly	19	19	24	19	21	18	20
not very understanding	-	5	10	13	11	9	6
other comment	10	6	11	8	7	5	10
Respondent thought the different aspects of care the person who died got from their general practitioner was:	%	%	%	%	%	%	%
excellent	52	48	36	44	36	42	35
good	32	32	33	26	39	33	35
fair	8	17	13	10	11	12	14
poor	3	3	8	14	9	6	8
no care	3	-	8	4	4	5	6
other comment	2	-	2	2	1	2	2
Number of people who died (=100%)	61	91	68	52	77	89	53

*People who spent all the last year of their lives in hospital and those for whom respondents did not make any assessments have been excluded when calculating percentages.

In the assessments, general practitioners in their forties tended to attract rather more criticisms than either younger or older general practitioners, but this difference only reached statistical significance over not being easy to talk to. Doctors in their late forties had larger lists than others: 40 per cent of them were in practices with average list sizes of 2,500 or more compared with 21 per cent of doctors aged 50 or more and 23 per cent of doctors under 45, but, as stated earlier, list size was not related to these assessments.

The proportion of women doctors fell from 24 per cent among those under 40, to 15 per cent of those in their forties and 6 per cent of those aged 50 or more. It seemed that women, like the younger doctors, were regarded as easier to talk to (92 per cent compared with 86 per cent of men) and to have more time to discuss things (86 per cent compared with 80 per cent), but neither of these differences was statistically significant.

Vocational training too was more common among the younger doctors: 78 per cent of those under 40 said they had been through a recognised vocational training scheme for general practice, 35 per cent of those in their forties, 14 per cent of those in their fifties but rising again to 38 per cent of those aged 60 or more. Those who had been trained under such a scheme were more often regarded as easy to talk to (92 per cent compared with 78 per cent) and their care of the person who died was less likely to be described as not very understanding (5 per cent compared with 11 per cent) or as "fair" or "poor" (14 per cent compared with 26 per cent). The difference in the proportion categorized as reluctant to visit, 9 per cent compared with 17 per cent, did not quite reach significance and the number of home visits reported for patients of the doctors in two groups was similar. An analysis confined to doctors aged 40 or more showed that the differences between the vocationally trained and the others remained and could not be just attributed to their age.

Nineteen per cent of the general practitioners were recorded in the Medical Register as being members or fellows of the Royal College of General Practitioners. There was no clear trend in this proportion with age or list size and the proportion was similar for men and women doctors. The care given to patients of College members was rated as excellent or good in 82 per cent of instances compared with 73 per cent of patients of non members, a difference which fell just short of statistical significance, and there were no significant differences in reported care although 27 per cent of College members were trainers compared with only 5 per cent of non members. It might be thought that trainers might be more highly rated by our respondents than other doctors but, as will be shown next, the only observed difference was in the opposite direction.

Ten per cent of the general practitioners in our sample were classified by the Department of Health as trainers, and the only significant difference between them and the others in our respondents' assessments was that more of the care given by trainers was described as not very understanding: 16 per cent compared with 7 per cent for other doctors. Possibly patients of doctors who were trainers were more often seen by trainees, locums or assistants. Certainly a relatively high proportion of the respondents for people whose doctor was a trainer felt it would have been better if they had seen fewer doctors: 32 per cent compared with 16 per cent of those who were not trainers, although the number of different doctors seen did not differ appreciably between the two groups (the average numbers were 2.3 and 2.1).

Comparisons were also made between doctors in the north and those south of the Bristol Wash line. There was no significant difference in the number of reported consultations and home visits nor in our respondents' assessments of care but more of the general practitioners in the south were in practices where the average list size was 2,500 or more: 32 per cent compared with 18 per cent in the north, and more of the doctors in the north qualified in Asia: 23 per cent compared with 9 per cent in the south.

An analysis by doctors in inner city areas, other metropolitan areas and county boroughs also showed no differences in the number of home visits or in respondents' assessments of care except that in the county boroughs doctors were more often thought not to have time to discuss things (by 18 per cent of the respondents compared with 10 per cent in other areas). Possibly people in county boroughs have higher expectations about this. Doctors in inner city areas tended to fall at the two extremes in relation to list size: 49 per cent of them compared with 36 per cent of other doctors had average list sizes under 2,000 and 10 per cent compared with two per cent had lists of 3,000 or more. A relatively high proportion of the inner city doctors were women, 24 per cent compared with 12 per cent in other areas, and the proportion who trained in Asia was 24 per cent in the inner city areas 15 per cent elsewhere, but this last difference did not quite reach statistical significance.

Looking at country of qualification, 75 per cent of the general practitioners qualified in Great Britain, 5 per cent in Ireland, 17 per cent in Asia and 3 per cent elsewhere. The numbers are only large enough to make comparisons between those qualifying in Great Britain and Asia. Comparatively few of those who qualified in Asia were under 40 (10 per cent compared with 35 per cent of those qualifying in Great Britain), members of the Royal College of General Practitioners (5 per cent compared with 25 per cent) or trainers (2 per cent compared with 12 per cent) but there were no significant differences between the two groups in relation to sex, size of list, nor in their views on whether they were able to give enough time to people who were dying. But people whose doctors qualified in Asia had fewer home visits (an average of 4.4 in the year before they died compared with 7.7 for those whose doctor qualified in G.B); they had fewer consultations altogether (8.0 compared with 10.6) but more consultations at the surgery (3.5 compared with 2.8). In addition, more of those qualifying in Asia were regarded as reluctant to visit: 24 per cent compared with 11 per cent of those qualifying in Britain. Another difference was that more of the doctors who qualified in Asia were described as not easy to talk to (19 per cent compared with 10 per cent). Also, their care of the person who died was more often felt to be "not very understanding" (16 per cent compared with 6 per cent) and as "poor" (16 per cent compared with 6 per cent). It is possible that some of the adverse assessments might result from racial prejudice, but the difference in the number of home visits in conjunction with the assessments about being reluctant to visit, suggest that people with doctors who qualified in Asia may be receiving less care from their general practitioners as well as having more communication problems than people whose doctor trained in Britain.

Conclusion

Although most of the people interviewed praised, or were satisfied with, the care given by general practitioners to the people who died, both the statistics and the quotations reveal some disconcerting inadequacies in this care. One problem is the unwillingness of some people to recognise or admit to their sickness and to seek help for it. Another is the difficulty some general practitioners have in coping with their own emotional reactions to death and dying, and, related to this, their inability to give appropriate care and support to people who are dying and their relatives. Only a quarter of the doctors had had any specific training in the care of the dying or management of bereavement and this study did not show any obvious benefits of this training to either the doctors themselves or their patients. Nevertheless half or more of the doctors thought it would be helpful to have further training in various aspects of this type of care.

A further problem for the general practitioners is lack of time and this was a particular difficulty for those with large numbers of patients on their lists. This was clear from the reports of the doctors and also from the smaller numbers of visits made to the people in our sample by doctors with larger lists.

Home visiting was much appreciated when it happened, but the lack of it, or its rarity, was the most frequent criticism made of the care given by general practitioners to people in the year before they died. A study of elderly people discharged from hospital also identified problems with home visiting as the commonest source of complaint (Williams and Fitton 1990). The decline in home visiting by general practitioners over the last quarter of a century (Cartwright and Anderson 1981) has come at a time when it is probably more needed by the housebound and seriously ill, as hospital stays have shortened and there is more and more emphasis on community care. The many comments and illustrations about the need for more home visiting do not suggest that visits by other members of the primary care team would be a satisfactory alternative to the doctor as it was usually medical observation and diagnosis that seemed to be needed. In one instance support was given almost entirely by the receptionist over the telephone, support which was much appreciated by the person at the time but which appeared quite inappropriate and inadequate in the long run. Selective home visiting might also overcome some of the reluctance of some elderly people to reveal the nature and extent of their ill health.

Gray in his 1977 James Mackenzie lecture (1978) emphasised the importance of home visiting by general practitioners. He was aware that this view was unpopular and contrary to trends in this country and across the Western World. He thought history might show him as a latter day Canute proverbially struggling to stem the tide. This study has shown some of the ill effects of that tide, but has also demonstrated the appreciation and gratitude of patients and relatives to those general practitioners who still stand out against that trend and give support and care in people's homes during the last year of their lives.

A possible way to help stem this tide is also demonstrated by this study: one way to audit care in general practice is by taking a sample of deaths and retrospectively looking at the care given in the months beforehand. If such studies were done at a local level they would reveal the good care as well as any gaps and inadequacies. Home visiting would be an important part of good care for this group of patients.

Notes

1. We did not ask these questions about the few (5 per cent) people who died suddenly when they were under 65 and we only asked respondents who had the same doctor as the person who died (51 per cent) and others who knew the doctor (27 per cent) about whether they thought the doctor was an easy person to talk to and had time to discuss things.

15 Community nurses

In 1969 the frequency, amount and nature of the care given by district nurses was described, using nurses' and relatives' accounts. Broader issues, such as the nurses' relationships with general practitioners and hospitals, and their views about community services were also described. The study raised questions about the adequacy of the district nursing service and the effectiveness of their relationship with medical and other community services.

As was shown in chapter one, there have been a number of changes in the nursing services available for care of the dying at home. An important development has been the rapid expansion of specialist terminal cancer teams, set up largely under the auspices of the MacMillan Fund, and associated with the hospice movement (see Table 1.1). Some research studies have focused on the work of these teams. Ward (1985) presents an account of the work of eight such teams showing that their approach to home care was largely advisory and supportive, rather than being devoted to practical nursing tasks, which were undertaken by relatives and district nurses. Ward concluded that overwork and isolation, as well as difficulties in gaining acceptance by professional colleagues such as general practitioners, were common problems faced by such nurses. Lunt and Yardley's (1986) study of 45 specialist teams found a similar emphasis on advice and support in the nurses' work. This study focused particularly on sources of stress and found that the most common source was the nurse's relationship with professional colleagues, particularly general practitioners. A fifth of the nurses said they did not get enough emotional support in their work and over half wanted more contact with other nurses in similar services.

The amount of research describing the work of such teams should not, however, obscure the fact that the majority of home nursing services for the terminally ill, let alone for those who die without a recognisably terminal illness, are still provided by district nurses. Yet recent research on the role of district nurses in this field has been small scale in Britain (Field 1989, MacDonald and MacNair 1986). With an ageing population it is important to assess the adequacy of a nursing service that is facing increased demand for care. In the present study relatives and nurses' accounts are drawn upon to both describe the care given and provide evaluations of adequacy. A particular focus is the nurses' own view of terminal care, especially about the stresses of providing emotional support to families. The relationships of nurses with other professionals, and their perceptions of the adequacy of support, are also explored.

The response

Two hundred and twenty four original respondents (35 per cent) reported visits from a nurse at home. In 56 cases more than one type of nurse was involved (for example, a person might have received visits from MacMillan nurses as well as district nurses). Provision was made in the questionnaire for the work of up to two types of nurse to be described. Thus original respondents described what happened in 280 nursing episodes. Table 15.1 gives the type of nurse involved at each stage of the project, showing that district nurses were somewhat over represented in the nurses' questionnaire returns.

Table 15.1
Type of nurse involved at each stage: original respondents, general views and specific patient questionnaires

	Reported by original respondents %	Answered general questionnaires %	Answered specific patient questionnaires %
District Nurse	70	85	79
Health Visitor	3	2	2
Nurse from hospice/ MacMillan	10	9	10
Nurse from general practice	9	0	5
Other	8	4	4
Total no. nurses' /episodes (N=100%)	280	92	113

There was no evidence that nurses judged by original respondents to be providing better quality nursing care were more likely to participate in the study than others. The response rates for both types of nurse questionnaire tended to be higher for people dying of cancer, those dying when comparatively young, those dying at home and those receiving more frequent and more long term nursing care. Cartwright and Seale (1990) report a more detailed account of response bias and other methodological issues of the study.

How adequate was the service?

Original respondents' perceptions of adequacy

One aspect of adequacy is the extent to which home nursing help was given to those who most needed it. Excluding those in the sample who were in hospital or other institutions all year, 12 per cent of the 308 people who did not receive nursing help at home were said by original respondents to have needed such help. Where nursing help was received, 22 per cent of the original respondents said that they would have preferred this to have been given more often. However, of all the people saying more nursing help was needed only a quarter had asked for it.

All these figures were similar to the 1969 study, where the same questions were asked, with no significant differences, suggesting that the service continues to meet needs at the same level as before. This is surprising in view of the fact that the pattern of visiting had changed since 1969, with people receiving less frequent visiting than in 1969, spread over a longer period of time (shown in Table 15.2).

The management by nurses of people with terminal cancer and their families has changed since 1969, with an increased emphasis on the education and support of family carers (Clench 1984, Saunders 1978, Simms 1984, Ward 1985). The success of this strategy may be the explanation for these figures. Alternatively, other services may have substituted for the community nurse. For example, in 1987 chiropodists were almost twice as likely to have visited those who needed help with cutting their toenails (40 per cent of those needing help as opposed to 23 per cent in 1969).

Nurses' views about the adequacy of the service in general

Superficially, the views of original respondents about adequacy were supported by the views of the nurses answering the general questionnaire. No change between the two time points was found in nurses' answers to a

Table 15.2
Visiting patterns of district nurses reported by original respondents: 1969 and 1987

	1969	1987
Period over which received help	%	%
< 1 week	21	12
1 week < 1 month	29	20
1 month < 3 months	20	18
3 months < 1 year	15	22
1 year +	15	28
No. of district nursing episodes (=100%)	229	174
How often visited (at most frequent)	%	%
Daily	56	41
Less than daily, more than weekly	23	38
Less than weekly	21	21
No. of district nursing episodes (=100%)	234	169

question asking "For patients who are dying would you describe the nursing service in your area as adequate, rather inadequate or very inadequate." In 1987 most of the nurses (76 per cent) saw the service as adequate and 23 per cent as rather inadequate, only one per cent seeing it as very inadequate, not significantly different from the figures in 1969. This is consistent with the small proportion of original respondents who had wanted more home nursing care, although the term "adequate" may well have been interpreted by nurses to mean other things as well.

Indeed, this global judgement by the nurses concealed a less favourable picture of adequacy in response to more specific questions. When asked on the general questionnaire whether there was "any sort of help or care which you feel that district nurses could give to dying patients that they are not giving at the moment," 48 per cent of the 92 nurses agreed. When then asked in an open ended question to specify the sort of help that was needed, and what stopped them from giving it, the most frequent reply (24 nurses) concerned the lack of time that district nurses had, due to a lack of resources. Some nurses commented further on what they would like to do with this time, the most frequent comment (made by 15) being that spending time talking or being with families and patients was what was needed. Related to this was the comment of ten more nurses who said that counselling was a service district nurses should be providing. For the most part, lack of resources was identified as the chief problem preventing this, although five identified a lack of training. Typical comments were: "Just more time really, to spend with them. There just isn't enough time"; "More time just chatting and giving confidence (we don't give it because of) staffing problems"; "Time to sit and be with them. (We don't give it because of) lack of time and lack of confidence in just sitting and listening."

When asked separately whether they felt "able to give enough time to patients who are dying," 58 per cent of the 92 nurses said they would like more time, and 42 per cent said they had enough time. These are similar proportions to district nurses' views in 1969, where nearly two thirds, when asked the same question, felt they would like more time.

Views about the adequacy of care for specific patients

The nurses, then, expressed a desire to spend more time with patients when commenting about their work as a whole on the general questionnaire. However when commenting on their care of particular individuals in the sample, the nurses answering the specific patient questionnaire were more ready to say they had had enough time. When asked "Did you feel you had enough time to do the things you needed to do when you visited," 75 per cent claimed that they had always had enough time, with only 4 per cent saying that they never did and the rest saying they sometimes did.

The discrepancy here between the nurses' general views and their accounts of specific episodes of care might be explained by an unwillingness to acknowledge difficulties when thinking of particular episodes of care. However original respondents in 81 per cent of the cases where nursing care was received said that nurses had in fact had enough time to do the things they did, which suggests a similar level of satisfaction with this aspect of nursing care to nurses' own assessments. It may be that in answering the general question about the need for more time nurses were reflecting on what they would like ideally to do, which went beyond both original respondents' expectations and nurses' actual views about what was necessary when considering their past practice.

However, when commenting reporting on the frequency of visiting there was evidence that nurses may have underestimated problems that were present. Most (88 per cent) of the nurses commenting on the care of individual patients in the specific patient questionnaire agreed that they had been able to visit "as often as, and at the times that, the patient needed" and few (12 per cent) felt that the relatives could have done with more nursing help. This compares with the 22 per cent of original respondents (reported earlier) who would have preferred more help. Further, when the accounts of both people could be compared, in 18 out of 28 cases over which nurses and respondents disagreed the original respondent felt more was needed, but the nurse did not.

When reflecting in general, then, on different aspects of the adequacy of the service, nurses tended to be in agreement with the relatives, friends and others who knew the people who died. Indeed, in terms of their generalised desire to spend more time with patients, nurses seem to be exceeding original respondents' expectations. When commenting on the care of individuals, however, the picture is less clear cut, with the findings suggesting that nurses' expectations may be somewhat lowered, even below those of original respondents as far as the frequency of visiting is concerned.

Further evidence about the variability of nurses' views was found in their answers to questions about the adequacy of the informal care provided to people by friends and relatives. When asked on the general questionnaire which, out of eight factors, was most likely to prevent more people being looked after in the community rather than hospital, the factor chosen most frequently by nurses was the absence of suitable relatives (45 per cent) followed by the unwillingness of relatives to look after people (21 per cent). However, when nurses in the specific patient questionnaire were asked "Would you say (the relatives) did not do enough, or did a reasonable amount, or had to do too much" none of the nurses were willing to say that relatives did not do enough. All of those answering this question said either that the relatives had done a reasonable amount (73 per cent) or had had to do too much (27 per cent). Thus there was a tendency to criticise relatives in general for this, but an unwillingness to point out individual cases.

It has long been recognised (Moser and Kalton 1971) that hypothetical or non personalised questions in surveys tend to elicit different responses compared to questions that require the respondent to choose between realistic options, or relate the response to their personal behaviour. Commentary on this (Moser and Kalton 1971, de Vaus 1990) normally implies that the more valid data comes from the second type of question. This may be the case with the data presented here, but if original respondent's views are taken as the yardstick to judge validity, there are indications, particularly concerning perceptions about the frequency of visiting, that nurses' views about adequacy were more hidden when discussing the care of individuals.

Referral and communication with other professionals

The 1969 study raised questions about the adequacy of nurses' communication with general practitioners and hospitals, particularly at the stage of patient referral. The results from 1987 allow comparison between the two time points to be made. Answers from the general questionnaire about the adequacy of communication are presented in Table 15.3. This shows that nurses were more critical of communication with hospitals than with general practitioners, but that communication with hospitals had improved since 1969, whereas that with general practitioners was not significantly different. However, nurses' fairly favourable ratings of communication when asked about it at this global level changed once more specific questions about the timing of referral and the information given at referral were asked.

Table 15.3
Adequacy of communication with hospitals and general practitioners judged by community nurses: 1969 and 1987

In caring for patients who are dying and who have been in hospital do you find communication with the hospital is generally

	1969	1987
	%	%
Adequate	32	46
Rather inadequate	33	38
Or very inadequate?	25	9
Other	9	7
Number of nurses (=100%)	506	92

In caring for patients who are dying do you find communication with their general practitioner is generally

	%	%
Adequate	81	76
Rather inadequate	14	12
Or very inadequate?	2	2
Other	3	11
Number of nurses (=100%)	506	92

Timing of referral

Referral was identified in the 1969 study as a stage at which communication issues were particularly important. The majority of referrals that brought the patients onto the records of the nurses answering the specific patient questionnaire in 1987 were from general practitioners (56 per cent) followed by hospital doctors (24 per cent). Although comparison over time of nurses' global ratings of communication with general practitioners showed no change, questioning about their feelings about referral showed a marked time change. In the general questionnaire nurses were asked "On the whole do you find that for patients who are dying general practitioners ask for nursing help earlier than necessary, not early enough or about the right time?" As with district nurses asked the same question in 1969, the number saying referral was too early was minimal (one case in 1987, 4 per cent in 1969), but the proportion saying that referral from the general practitioner, on the whole, was not early enough had risen from 14 per cent of district nurses in 1969 to 48 per cent of nurses in 1987. This may reflect changes in general practitioners' behaviour, or it may reflect a changed awareness in nurses about what can be done for patients and their families if early contact is made. The increased emphasis on patient and family education in self care (noted earlier) may also be responsible for such a change in awareness.

Consistent with this are nurses' views on the advantages of early referral, which were described by ten nurses in qualitative comments from the general questionnaire. Fairly typical was a district nurse who said: "If we know about something (early enough) we can build up a relationship but if you go in late things are at a crisis pitch by the time you get there and they haven't got the confidence. Its the family as well." Another described a case of late referral:

> A few months back there was a lady with a breast with bony secondaries and the GP only referred her to us when she became constipated because of the medication. She was in her seventies and they weren't receiving any help apart from the GP visiting...by the time we got involved the family was at screaming pitch. We were able to arrange a home help, social worker and Macmillan nurse but had this been done earlier there would have been a better relationship between the family and the nursing staff.

Nurses describing episodes of care on the specific patient questionnaire were asked "Do you feel the service was asked for at the right time, or that it would have been appropriate to ask for it earlier or later?" In view of the feeling expressed on the general questionnaire by nearly half the nurses that referral from general practitioners was, on the whole, not early enough, it is instructive to note that this problem was identified by nurses in only 29 per cent of the cases where nurses were asked to comment on the care of specific individuals in the sample, with 70 per cent feeling that referral had occurred at the right time. Further, when asked to comment on how earlier referral would have helped, the relief of physical symptoms was accorded priority in equal, if not greater, frequency to the need to build a good relationship with family members. Thus, ten nurses mentioned the relief of physical problems: "He had MS, was disabled and had a gangrenous, diseased penis. He may not have died if (there had been) earlier care"; "She had massive swollen legs with oedema that were weeping...she was quite a poorly lady. Maybe I'd have been able to make her more comfortable than she was if we'd been called in earlier." Seven felt the relationship with the patient or family had suffered: "To build up a relationship before he became so poorly...I felt his wife could have done with more support. We were only involved for about a week."

As with their judgements of the adequacy of the nursing service, it appears that the nurses had higher expectations when asked about referral in general than when considering specific episodes of patient care. This may be associated with an increased awareness of the need to establish supportive relationships with patients and their families early on, although the physical care aspects of nursing work seemed equally vivid when nurses contemplated specific episodes of care. At the same time, dissatisfaction with the timing of referral, particularly that from general practitioners, was more widespread than might initially have been expected from the global ratings about the adequacy of communication (Table 15.3).

Information at referral

Whether referral had increasingly become too late or not, nurses' views about the general adequacy of information given them at referral, whether from general practitioners, hospitals or other sources, had not changed since 1969. Here again, this aspect of nurses' relationship with other professionals showed a higher level of dissatisfaction than in their initial, global rating of the adequacy of communication. When asked on the general questionnaire "When patients are referred to you for home nursing care would you, in general, describe the information you get as adequate, rather inadequate or very inadequate?" 59 per cent of the 92 nurses said rather or very inadequate.

When those who said this were asked "What sort of things would you like to have more information about?" most commonly mentioned was a need to know more about the patient's medical condition at referral. Fifteen nurses said they often needed to know the diagnosis or prognosis, 13 wanted more about the general medical history, and seven identified specific details that were often absent, such as details about which medications were to be taken by the patient, or the type of dressings needed. The level of dependency was mentioned by eight. The next most commonly mentioned information need was for information about the family composition and their degree of participation in care, mentioned by 16. Comments include: "We always have to ring round for more information, ie: if it's terminal, who knows the diagnosis and how much the patient knows. We have to play it by ear. I've never yet put my foot in it but there's always a chance"; "We get what (the patient) was in (hospital) for but would like more about their home circumstances and general condition. You get "can manage" ticked and find the person is immobile and the toilet is upstairs."

The issue exemplified by the first of these comments concerns knowing what the family knew about the diagnosis or prognosis, mentioned by 11 nurses. As communication and awareness were particular areas of concern in the study (see chapter three) nurses were asked a separate question about this on the general questionnaire: "When a terminally ill patient is referred to you do you know what the patient has been told about the prognosis always, usually, occasionally or never?" A large proportion (44 per cent) said that they only occasionally knew, with a further 2 per cent saying they never knew, the rest saying always (13 per cent) or usually (41 per cent). In fact, 49 per cent of the nurses answering the specific patient questionnaire said they "knew what the patient had been told about his/her prognosis" at the first visit.

Again, what the nurses said when reflecting on the general adequacy of information at referral can be compared with their views concerning individual patients. Once again, nurses were less willing to identify problems when answering about specific patients they had seen. All the nurses were asked whether, at the first visit, "the information you had been given before you went was adequate, rather inadequate or very inadequate." Most felt that is was adequate (73 per cent) with only 25 per cent saying that it was rather or very inadequate. This compares with the 59 per cent (reported earlier) who reported on their general questionnaire that information at this stage was, in general, not adequate.

Those who said that information about specific patients was inadequate were asked in what way this was so. Here, the needs identified were similar to those identified by nurses on the general questionnaire. The most frequent comments, made by 11, specified information about the clinical condition or treatment that had been missing. For example: "I had to find out myself that she had a bladder infection and that the GP wanted her catheterised." Eight described what they had been told, stressing the paucity of information of any sort: "I found him in a poor state, confused and agitated, but his wife was desperate to get him home. I was not given a lot of information at all, just the diagnosis. I didn't expect to find him so bad"; "All I got was name, address and request for a bath. I found out everything about him when I visited...then I found he had a chronic chest infection. I think we should generally be given more information." Five others wanted to know more about the home circumstances or patient's psychological state: "I was unprepared for the total squalor, that it was a condemned building and that there was livestock everywhere (dogs and cats). The Environmental Health said they had never seen so many dogs. It stunk. Cat's excrement everywhere. Later when she had diarrhoea there was her urine and excrement everywhere. She just went in her chair"; "I didn't know he was very shy and reserved with females. I didn't know the family either."

Pain control

Simms (1984) describes a number of instances of nurses specialising in terminal care feeling critical of standards of pain control by general practitioners. Indeed, responsibility for pain control has been identified by Mor (1987) as a key area for inter professional boundary disputes in terminal care. In the light of this, nurses in the 1987 study were asked about sources of problems with pain control to see whether general practitioners were identified.

As described in chapter thirteen, over a third of the 92 nurses felt that pain could be controlled satisfactorily in more patients than was in fact the case. When asked why 18 nurses mentioned the poor prescribing practices or lack of knowledge of general practitioners and 15 nurses mentioned poor compliance by patients. This was compounded, in the view of seven nurses, by difficulty in knowing the level of pain present, either because of the stoicism of some people, or that the pain being reported was really a reflection of the patients' fear. Comments that illustrate these themes are as follows: "Sometimes it's the patients' or relatives' reluctance to take medication. Sometimes it's not prescribed in big enough doses. Sometimes the GPs are not familiar with modern analgesics. They tend to use a certain drug and stick with it"; "Sometimes it's a reluctance of GPs to prescribe narcotics. Also the patients think because they've got cancer they're going to have pain."

The existence of problems with general practitioners in the area of pain control seem to be supported, then, by nurses' views in the 1987 survey. On this, as on other aspects of the findings which show nurses being critical of general practitioners, it is important not to take the nurses' views purely at face value. The results show that nurses' views on a number of topics vary according to whether they are considering the service in general, or specific episodes of care.

Nurses' stress, support and training needs

Half of the nurses interviewed for the general questionnaire said that they found it difficult or rather difficult coping with the emotional distress of terminally ill patients and their relatives. Thirty seven per cent found their own reactions to death and dying difficult or rather difficult to cope with and 73 per cent said they found it more stressful looking after people who were dying than caring for other patients. When asked in an open ended question why they found it stressful, the most common response was to say that these were situations where they became emotionally involved (said by 40 nurses). Another common response, sometimes in conjunction with the above, was that the distress of the patient's family was an important factor. Typical comments were: "You've also got the relatives to deal with as well, and you get attached to them if you are going in every day, and it does affect you emotionally. You get to know them and they get quite close to you really. You wouldn't be human if you weren't affected"; "You become very involved, see them every day and have to counsel patients and family. You have to care for the whole family unit." Nine nurses said that knowing that death would be the outcome rather than recovery was in itself stressful: "Because of knowing they are going to die. It's never really a happy situation. It's always more satisfying to see a patient get better." Six commented that it was more difficult if it was a young person dying, and five said that where the person was not supposed to know they were dying it was more stressful.

Although most (85 per cent) of the nurses said that the amount of contact they had with others in the field was adequate, fewer (61 per cent) said they got as much help and support as they needed. Thirty six per cent said they did not get enough help and support. When asked to identify from whom they got help and support the most frequently mentioned people were other nursing colleagues (92 per cent) followed by family and friends (64 per cent), a general practitioner (53 per cent) and a nursing manager (37 per cent). Sixteen per cent said that they found one or more general practitioners unhelpful.

Religious faith seemed to help many of the nurses in their work with the dying. Forty one per cent said they had a strong religious faith and a further 47 per cent had some. Of these, 75 per cent said that they found it helpful in their work. Seventy four per cent of the nurses said they believed in a life after death. This can be compared with only 53 per cent of original respondents who believed this.

Fifty five per cent of the nurses had had some form of training in terminal care. Of these, all but three found it very or fairly helpful. All but six of the 92 nurses answering the general questionnaire felt that it would be helpful to have further training relating to terminal care, with the management of pain being the most popular area of training need (82 per cent) followed by bereavement counselling (78 per cent), relief of nausea and vomiting (71 per cent), communicating with dying patients (67 per cent) and control of breathlessness (65 per cent).

Conclusion

Original respondents' perceptions of the adequacy of domiciliary nursing show little change between 1969 and 1987, measured in terms of whether help was given where needed. Overall the vast majority of these respondents were satisfied with the amount of help received. It is tempting to consider how the nursing service given to this group might have improved in adequacy had resources in 1987 been sufficient to maintain the frequency of visiting that there was in 1969. However, changes in the management of patients and their families, with a greater stress on a "hands off" supportive and educational role could explain the findings.

At the same time, it is important to recognise that this is only one aspect of adequacy, and that the expectations of the relatives, friends and others who acted as respondents in this part of the survey need not be taken as the bench mark for setting standards. Indeed, there was evidence that the nurses themselves had higher expectations of the service than original respondents in some areas, particularly in the widespread desire to spend more time with patients and families in order to provide emotional rather than solely practical support.

A marked feature of the findings from the two nurses' questionnaires was the difference in their views according to whether nurses were considering the nursing service for the dying generally, or whether they were considering the care of individual patients. On the whole, nurses were more willing to be critical of the service in general than of the standards they achieved in practice. With regard to the frequency and amount of visiting for each patient, and this is something that has declined since 1969, nurses were in danger of having even lower standards than original respondents, who were somewhat more likely to see problems with this than the nurses themselves.

How can we reconcile the fact that nurses were able to say on the one hand that in general they needed more time to spend with families, and on the other that enough time was available for the particular patients they were asked about in the survey? A similar issue is raised by the finding that the nurses were willing to criticise relatives in general for not doing enough for patients, yet could not point to a single case where this had occurred when commenting on the care of particular individuals. Nurses appear to be unwilling to be critical either of themselves or family members when considering individual episodes of care.

One possibility is that nurses were reflecting the ideals they had for the service when making their general comments, whereas when faced with the practical realities of patient care these ideals were easy to forget. Another is that it was difficult for a nurse to admit that an episode of care for which he or she had been responsible was not of an adequate standard, as such a conclusion might just as well have implications for the nurses' professional competence as for the under resourcing of the service. Neither of these, however, account for the discrepancy over their views on relatives' willingness to care. In different contexts people bring different frames of reference to bear (Hammersley and Atkinson 1983). The widely held view that the quality of family support for the elderly has declined over the years may have influenced nurses' views here, contrary though it was to their actual experience of working with families. (The care that was given by family and friends is reported in chapter five).

A marked difference from 1969 is that nurses in 1987 were more than three times as likely to complain of late referral of patients by general practitioners. Once again, nurses were somewhat less likely to identify this as a problem when describing the care of individual patients. The change since 1969 may well reflect heightened expectations, particularly those concerning the development of a supportive role for families, rather than a changed referral pattern. Certainly the nurses in 1987 expressed a strong desire to spend more time with patients and relatives, building up a relationship and giving emotional support rather than just doing physical tasks, although again the physical realities of actual patient care seemed equally, if not more, important when contemplating actual episodes of care.

If there had been changes towards later referral, these will largely have arisen from general practitioners' actions as most referrals were from this source. There were also indications that some nurses were critical of general practitioners' prescribing practices in relation to pain control, supporting the findings of other studies in this field (Simms 1984).

The findings also show that nurses have to cope with a substantial amount of stress arising from their emotional involvement with families where a person is dying. They may feel a lack of control over important determinants of distress, such as drug doses, or telling the prognosis, or arriving early enough in the course of disease. This may be responsible for resentful feelings towards general practitioners, who have more control over these matters, but less daily involvement. What is not clear from these findings, however, is whether giving nurses more control over such decisions would result in a reduction in stress for nurses. Providing nursing help for people who are dying may be stressful under any circumstances.

In describing the emotional demands and constraints of their work with dying people, the nurses emphasised their need for more time to spend with such people and their families. Clearly, perceptions of the nursing service as overstretched were not confined to nurses, but were shared by at least a small proportion of relatives, and others may have tailored their expression of need to this constraint. Nurses in general wanted time to spend talking with patients and families, even though they found it harder to admit the need when discussing individual patient care. Caring for the dying was perceived as emotionally stressful, in large part because of the distress of family members as well as patients. The nurses for the most part were drawn into this distress. Creating a better environment for patient care in the home, is clearly dependent not just on training, the attitudes or social skills of nurses, or the extent of their rights to make decisions about care, important though these things are, but in having the time to talk.

16 The relationship between professionals

In the last year of life most people need a lot of care. Many receive this from both professionals and non professionals, from doctors in the community and in hospitals, and from nurses. The relationships between people providing these different sources of help affects the adequacy, effectiveness and humanity of care during this period. It is often a particularly poignant time for the people themselves and a memorable one for the relatives who live on.

This chapter is about the relationship between three professional groups: community nurses, general practitioners and hospital consultants. It also looks at the views and experiences of these three groups concerning specialist domiciliary terminal care services, such as MacMillan nursing teams.

General practitioners and hospitals

The great majority of general practitioners, 84 per cent, thought there was adequate consultation between them and hospital medical staff over the admission of patients. But only 22 per cent thought this about consultation over discharge, the majority, 76 per cent, being critical over this. Most of the criticisms related to delays. Other comments were that general practitioners were sometimes not told when a patient had died, that junior doctors did not understand the problems of general practice and that a better understanding of the problems of the ill patient who was coping alone was needed by the hospital team.

General practitioners were asked whether when a patient had a terminal illness diagnosed at the hospital the hospital staff let them know what, if anything, they had told the patient. Only 4 per cent said they always did, 41 per cent usually, 47 per cent occasionally and 8 per cent said it never happened. A number pointed out that it should be always.

Hospital consultants, like general practitioners, thought that adequate consultation happened more often over admissions (75 per cent) than over discharge (57 per cent), but fewer consultants than general practitioners thought consultation over discharge was inadequate. Presumably they are not so aware of, or affected by, any delays in the despatch of discharge letters.

Domiciliary consultations, when hospital consultants visit patients in their homes at the request of general practitioners, are a potential meeting ground between these two groups of professionals and at these consultations decisions are often made about hospital admission or care in the community. Both these groups of doctors were asked whether they considered the arrangements for domiciliary consultations to be satisfactory or not. The majority of general practitioners, 85 per cent, regarded them as satisfactory; rather fewer consultants, 76 per cent.

The few criticisms made by the general practitioners focused on difficulties and delays in arranging such consultations and particularly in making them joint consultations. One saw them as "a racket to by pass waiting times". Several commented that they were now largely confined to two disciplines, geriatrics and psychiatry. Consultants too were unhappy about the numbers of domiciliary consultations at which general practitioners were not present. They were also critical of the way such visits were arranged, their use for securing admission and the selection of patients for domiciliary consultation: "It would be better if I could meet with the general practitioner more often, but time is usually too pressed to allow precise time tabling"; "Generally domiciliary visits not used in optimum way. Request often from receptionists to my secretary. I would prefer GP to speak to me direct" (Consultant in general medicine); "Sometimes it's a short cut to an out patient appointment, sometimes to admission, but admission would be given if asked for in the first place" (Consultant in geriatric medicine); "Lack of proper discussion and referral by GPs. My personal experience is that 90 per cent are inappropriate. An enormous manpower wastage" (General physician).

Others were critical of general practitioners for not asking for more domiciliary consultations: "A lot of GPs are good. They call for domiciliaries for assessments, but a lot just want me to admit the patient. They say there is no point in a domiciliary visit, but I think there is. It gives me a picture of the social background and that is most important" (Consultant in geriatrics).

This last comment was from a geriatrician who estimated that he had done between 100 and 120 domiciliary visits to patients who were dying in the previous year. Only 2 per cent of the consultants estimated that they had done 90 or more, 47 per cent had done none, 32 per cent one to four, 10 per cent five to nine and 9 per cent ten or more. Satisfaction with the arrangements was unrelated to the number of such visits they had made to patients who were dying. Comparatively few of those specialising in geriatrics or psychogeriatrics had not made any domiciliary consultations to patients who were dying in the last year (20 per cent compared with 55 per cent of those in other specialties) and all but one of the consultants who had done ten or more such visits specialised in geriatrics, psychogeriatrics, general medicine, terminal palliative or hospice care. (The exception was a surgeon who estimated that he had done 12 such visits).

General practitioners were asked to estimate how many domiciliary consultations, if any, they had asked for in the last 12 months for patients who were dying. Almost two fifths (39 per cent), said none, almost half (47 per cent), one to four, 7 per cent five to nine and 7 per cent ten or more. Again satisfaction with arrangements was not related to the number they had requested, although one who was dissatisfied commented that there was no point in asking for any.

Another issue explored was general practitioners' access to NHS beds where they retained full responsibility for treatment and to which they could admit patients for terminal care. Just over a fifth of general practitioners (22 per cent), said they had such beds; 61 per cent of those without any said they would like to have some and a similar proportion, 65 per cent, of those with access to some beds wanted more.

General practitioners and community nurses

Most general practitioners (86 per cent), found the district nursing service very helpful for patients who were dying; nearly all the others (13 per cent), described the service as "fairly helpful." Even so two fifths wanted to see some changes in the way the district nursing service was organised. More night cover and more staff were the most frequently mentioned changes needed. Several doctors wanted more or closer practice attachments and some thought that district nurses should be employed by the Family Practitioner Committee. Some other suggestions were: "There are no arrangements for nurses to stay at a house for long periods. This can only be arranged privately at present"; "In general too many nurses are involved to give the intimate care needed"; "A quicker response to needs, e.g. for incontinence pads"; "Ability to give injections (when needed) more frequently."

The majority of general practitioners, 86 per cent, indicated that if a patient needed just nursing care that relatives were able and prepared to give they still tended to ask the district nurse to visit. They said they did this mainly so that the nurses could give advice and support, "to establish a contact which may be useful to patient and relatives later" and to "demonstrate availability." Nevertheless, as reported in chapter fifteen, almost half the community nurses (48 per cent), said that on the whole general practitioners did not ask for nursing help early enough for people who were dying and only one said that they asked for help earlier than was necessary. As indicated in the last chapter (Table 15.3) some nurses felt critical of communication with general practitioners. One said: "We have extremes. We have GPs who are really caring and who visit patients frequently, and others who don't visit unless asked and don't speak to us at all. We make them verbalise, but if they can get away with a name and address only they do."

Community nurses and hospital consultants

As shown in Table 15.3 community nurses were more likely to be critical about communications with hospitals than with general practitioners. Comments from two who described it as "rather inadequate" were: "I have to initiate communication with the hospital but the tone of their response often suggests that we're two separate teams, not one"; "Sometimes (communication) non existent, but I can appreciate the problems hospitals have and it's my job to seek information." One who thought it "very inadequate" said: "The hospitals tend to be a law unto themselves, to work in isolation and not to give information to community services unless pushed." Several of those who said it was adequate indicated that the initiative often came from the nurses: "Because you make a point of doing it yourself if you're not happy."

Hospital consultants were asked whether they would describe the district nursing service in their area as adequate, rather inadequate or very inadequate. One in eight said they did not know. Among the others 54 per cent thought it adequate, 42 per cent rather inadequate and 4 per cent very inadequate. The picture that emerged from their comments was of understaffing and inadequate evening and night cover:"Too few, inadequate 24 hour and seven day a week servicing (which is) vital if community care is to be a reality rather than a financial sleight of hand"; "Adequate, but grossly overworked at times." There were some comments on the results of the inadequacies: "This is the main reason why even if the patient and the family want the terminally ill to be nursed at home, they have to be admitted to hospital."

Specialist domiciliary terminal care services

Around three quarters of the general practitioners, hospital consultants and community nurses reported that there were some home nurses specialising in terminal care in their area, and around two thirds said that specialist domiciliary medical advice on symptom relief for terminal care was available. General practitioners seemed less likely than either hospital consultants or community nurses to want these specialist services introduced if they were not available, or extended if they were (Table 16.1). In addition, when general practitioners and hospital consultants were asked whether they thought domiciliary nursing services specialising in terminal care were (if they had them), or could be (if they did not), very helpful, fairly helpful or not helpful, hospital consultants more often than general practitioners thought they were or would be very helpful, 81 per cent compared with 62 per cent.

Table 16.1
Availability of specialist domiciliary services and views on whether they should be introduced or extended*

Home nurses specialising in terminal care

	Available			Want extended or introduced		
	GPs	Consultants	Nurses	GPs	Consultants	Nurses
	%	%	%	%	%	%
	77	76	88	26	43	36
	(240)	(188)	(91)	(240)	(160)	(90)

Domiciliary specialist medical advice on symptom relief for terminal care

	Available			Want extended or introduced		
	GPs	Consultants	Nurses	GPs	Consultants	Nurses
	%	%	%	%	%	%
	62	68	72	23	31	34
	(232)	(180)	(92)	(232)	(153)	(89)

*The figures in brackets are the numbers on which percentages are based (=100%). Small proportions (between none and 5 per cent of community nurses and general practitioners did not answer these questions, larger proportions of consultants (between 11 per cent and 27 per cent).

Comments from the general practitioners indicate why 29 per cent of them thought the service was or would be only fairly helpful: "They won't help with physical nursing so the district nurses have to go in anyway"; "We ask for their help for most patients dying at home and they're very supportive. However only 9-5 Mondays to Fridays"; "They haven't quite got the knack of liaising with the GP. A bit over self confident at times. Apt to rush in before they know the situation."

Among the general practitioners who said they had a domiciliary specialist nursing service available in their area 67 per cent found it very helpful, but only 47 per cent of those without such a service thought it would be. Consultants with and without the service were equally convinced of its helpfulness.

Some consultants were aware of the potential conflict between general practitioners and specialist home nursing services: "The service falls down because it is not properly integrated. GPs seem unhappy." Others reiterated the familiar problem: "There are too few to be of any real use to patients and their families." Whereas 56 per cent of the consultants thought it would be better for home nurses specialising in terminal care to be attached to a hospice (47 per cent) or hospital (9 per cent) and only 16 per cent thought it would be best if they were part of the district nursing service, the general practitioners were almost equally divided in their preference for this last option (40 per cent) and attachment to a hospice (36 per cent) or hospital (5 per cent). Some of the reasons general practitioners gave for preferring them to be part of the district nursing service were: "Important, so they liaise with attached DNs who do the day to day care"; "Being part of the DN services there will be a better liaison between GP and nursing service." Reasons for preferring hospital attachment were both positive and negative: "Best to have them attached to the district hospital so that if admission is required it is much easier to arrange"; "Our district nursing service is rather authoritarian and tends to restrict the activity allowed to nurses. Should be independent of this." Some consultants also saw advantages in arranging admission if the specialist nurses were attached to a hospital. A number attached more importance to the outcome than to the organization: "Main thing is they are available and we know how to find them"; "I don't think it matters as long as it's good." One consultant who favoured attachment to a hospice made a different point: "They (nurses) need a base for emotional support and I feel a hospice is the right one."

Hospital consultants were also more enthusiastic than general practitioners about domiciliary specialist medical advice on symptom relief. The proportions who thought it would or could be very helpful were two thirds of the hospital doctors, half the general practitioners. Both general practitioners and hospital consultants were more convinced of the helpfulness of this service if it was available in their area (Table 16.2). Some consultants had reservations: "Good all round medical and nursing education would be better"; "Those GPs who would need the help most are less likely to ask for it"; "Probably unnecessary if GPs are good." A number of general practitioners also felt they should be able to cope without specialist help: "GPs can and should learn how to do this adequately. Courses are available." Others found the service "well established and helpful." General practitioners were more likely to feel the specialist service would be very helpful if they themselves wanted further training in pain management: 60 per cent compared with 37 per cent of those who did not want further training in this.

The community nurses who were not themselves specialists in the care of the dying were asked whether they had had any contact with nurses specialising in the care of the dying. Nine tenths had had some contact, mainly with specialist nurses who were part of the district nursing service (37 per cent) or attached to hospices (36 per cent). (The others had a variety of affiliations). Seventy nine per cent of those who had had some contact with specialist nurses said they had found them very helpful, 13 per cent fairly helpful, 3 per cent not helpful, the rest making other comments. The assessments were similar whether the specialist nurses were attached to a hospital or hospice or were part of the district nursing service. Many of the comments were enthusiastic: "Fantastic girls. Very supportive to us and to patients. Expertise is wonderful." Their admiration was sometimes enforced by the feeling or recognition of their own reluctance or inability to do that type of work: "Marvellous, brilliant. I don't think I could cope with it."

Table 16.2
Views on helpfulness of specialist domiciliary advice on symptom relief for terminal care by whether service available in their area[*]

		The proportions thinking service was or would be very helpful	
		General practitioners	Hospital consultants
Service available	Yes	56% (147)	74% (122)
in their area	No	38% (86)	52% (56)
All doctors[a]		49% (244)	66% (204)

[*]Figures in brackets are the numbers on which the percentages are based (=100%). [a]Includes the 11 general practitioners (5 per cent) and 26 (13 per cent) consultants who did not know if the service was available in their area.

While specialist nurses were sometimes seen as supporting the district nurses as well as patients and relatives, not all district nurses welcomed them: "They don't do much really. Just monitor pain relief. We do all the nursing and it causes a bit of resentment sometimes."

A third of the non specialist community nurses said they would like to see some changes in the way the specialist nursing service was organised and there were a number of other comments and suggestions. Again a need for more nurses and for more time were the most frequent comments. The different reactions indicate that nurses involved in the specialist service were resolving the conflict between looking after a few patients well, or more patients less well, in different ways. "There aren't enough of them. They can't limit themselves to time so they can only see so many"; "I'd like to see them visiting more often, as they did originally, rather than ringing patients, but they seem too busy now." Some wanted more contact with them. Others wanted better co-ordination between the district nursing and specialist service and another suggestion was that district nurses should do more of this work: "More of us to be trained." Indeed, 86 per cent of the district nurses said they would find it helpful to have further training in the management of pain; rather fewer (65 per cent) thought this about training in communication with dying patients. Seven out of the nine nurses specialising in the care of the dying also thought it would be helpful to have more training in both these fields. All of them felt they had good relationships with the other home nurses in their area.

Conclusion

The inadequate communication between general practitioners and hospitals over discharge is particularly serious for people in the last year of their lives as people are often admitted more than once during this time (see chapter ten) and they are likely to need supportive services at home when they are discharged. The problem is not simply related to delays: that so few consultants apparently let general practitioners know what they have told patients when they make a diagnosis of a terminal illness seems shocking. Hospital staff were also criticised by community nurses over their communications relatively frequently. It would seem that improvements are needed over both the content and the organization of communication from hospitals.

The image of the hospital consultant in an ivory tower, suggested by the comments of some community nurses, was reinforced by the observation that one in eight consultants said they did not know whether the community services in their area were adequate or not.

Over three tenths of the general practitioners wanted some or more NHS beds where they could retain full responsibility for treatment and to which they could admit patients for terminal care. An increase in such beds might ease the problems of arranging hospital admission for both young and old patients who needed long term care which most general practitioners reported some difficulty with. It could also reduce the over treatment of terminally ill patients in hospital which two fifths of the general practitioners thought occurred at least fairly often (see chapter thirteen).

The two professional groups working in the community, general practitioners and community nurses, were generally appreciative of each other and understanding of each other's problems. When general practitioners were critical of the district nursing service they often did not blame the nurses. One wrote: "We are terribly short of community nursing services. The patients don't get *cared for*. They get some things done to them but all at top speed. There is no time to show relatives what to do. No time to think what is going on. *It isn't the nurse's fault.* Sometimes there are three nurses to be shared among 20,000 patients!"

As many general practitioners feel the community nursing service is overstretched they may be reluctant to add to their workload by early referral, even though they recognise that as desirable. But it is a further indication of the large unmet need for nursing care at home that nearly half the nurses felt that general practitioners did not ask for nurses' help early enough for people who were dying.

General practitioners were rather less enthusiastic than the other two professional groups about specialist medical or nursing domiciliary terminal care. Another study found that most nurses in terminal care reported at least some quite serious problems in their relationship with local doctors, both general practitioners and hospital doctors, although nearly all stressed that these were a difficult minority and that most doctors were sympathetic and willing to learn about terminal care (Simms 1984). Others have commented on an attitude among general practitioners to the hospice movement, to hospital consultants and to "counselling" by other professionals which borders on antipathy (Aldridge 1987).

Clearly the usefulness and acceptability of specialist medical and nursing care are complex issues, depending on the skills and interests of both specialist and non specialist carers, the willingness of all parties to co-operate and the organization to facilitate this co-operation. It is encouraging that for the most part doctors were more convinced of the usefulness of the specialist services when they had some experience of the service.

17 Conclusion

We are now in a position to assess the significance of the changes that have occurred since 1969 in people's experience of the last year of life, and to consider prospects for the future. In this concluding chapter we draw together some of the main themes of the book and consider the significance of the findings for the different people involved in providing care.

The effect of demographic change

The increase in longevity and changes in the household structure of the elderly in Britain outlined in chapter one were reflected in the experiences of the people in the study. Increases in the proportions living alone (Table 2.2) or in institutional care (Table 2.3) were experienced particularly by women, who frequently had cared for a dying spouse, since spouses (predominantly wives) were the people most likely to bear the brunt of care in 1987 (chapter five). Spouses were also most likely to find adjustment to bereavement difficult (chapter five, Table 5.4). The ageing of the population was also reflected in the greater prevalence of certain long term symptoms, notably mental confusion, depression and incontinence (chapter two).

As Arber and Ginn (1991) have noted, the quality of life of the elderly is influenced by both access to the resource of informal care, and by the availability of financial resources. The decline in the availability of informal care was described in chapter five, where it was reported that in 1969 an average of three relatives or friends looked after each person in the sample, this declining to two by 1987. Chapter six highlighted the important role which money can play in supporting a good quality of life.

Given this picture of increasing need and decreasing informal resources, the role of formal services in supporting those in their last year of life assumes greater importance. This affects both the comfort of those who are dying, and the burden and stress of caring. Providing support and respite for carers is a role that can be played by community services, and an important means by which a policy of maintaining care for people in their own homes can be successfully pursued.

Day care clearly plays a role here, as it did for nine per cent of the people who died in 1987. However, the lack of attractiveness of such care in the eyes of some old people is reflected in the finding that respondents for a further 11 per cent said that such care would have been beneficial, but most of these people had not wanted to go to such a centre. There was evidence of some conflict between the wishes of those needing care to be looked after by people close to them and the needs of their carers for some respite from these demands. Initiatives in day care that involve informal carers themselves in providing such care might make it more acceptable to the people needing such care and could possibly relieve the loneliness and responsibility of the carers looking after people on their own.

General practice

National statistics (Table 1.3) show an increase between 1969 and 1987 in the numbers of people aged 75 and over per general practitioner. This is in spite of a better ratio of general practitioners to the population as a whole. As well as the move towards group practices, the other major change which official statistics show in general practice is the decline in home visiting, particularly to the elderly (Table 1.4).

This last change was the one that attracted the most criticisms from respondents (chapter fourteen), many more of whom in 1987, compared to 1969, identified the lack of home visiting by general practitioners as a problem. Although there were grumbles about seeing too many different doctors, this was not as important an issue as home visiting, which was of particularly concern for those who lived alone, who tended to get fewer such visits. On a more positive note, though, is the finding that more general practitioners in 1987 were found to be easy to talk to, and to have time to discuss things (chapter two).

It was noted in the conclusion to chapter fourteen that a call for more home visiting was likened by the senior member of the Royal College of General Practitioners who made it (Gray 1978) to Canute's appeal to the tide. However, if older housebound people are to be cared for satisfactorily in the community some way must be found to give them better access to the care they need. More carefully targeted home visiting by general practitioners is one solution. Some other possible options are discussed below.

Domiciliary nursing services

The decline in the number of district nurses per head of the elderly population (Table 1.5) was reflected in the less frequent visits which district nurses made in 1987 to those in the last year of life (chapter fifteen, Table 15.2). Although national statistics suggest that a greater proportion of the elderly were treated in 1987 than before (Table 1.5) this was not reflected in the experience of the sample, as a similar proportion as in 1969 received treatment from district nurses (chapter two). In spite of a more thinly stretched service, however, respondents' perceptions of unmet need for such care was at similar levels to 1969. In chapter fifteen it was suggested that this might be due to other services filling the gaps; the home help and chiropody services had doubled their coverage since 1969 (reported in chapters two and fifteen). However, the three groups of professionals surveyed, general practitioners, hospital consultants and community nurses, were all more likely to identify a need for more home help services than district nursing services (Table 13.2) and relatives, too, commonly identified a need for more help at home, particularly for those living alone (chapter thirteen).

Another explanation for the lack of increase in dissatisfaction with coverage by community nurses may have been successful management of care by advising and supporting informal carers to a greater extent than in the past. People aged 85 and over, though, who were more likely than others to be living alone, were judged to have more unmet need for domiciliary nursing services than others (chapter seven).

In general the 1987 study depicts a nursing service that is hard pressed to keep up with demands. The nurses themselves often felt a need to spend more time with patients and their families, and there was a widespread perception amongst the three groups of professionals involved that an extension of night sitting or night nursing services would be valuable (Table 13.3).

Nurses in 1987 were considerably more likely than in 1969 to complain of late referral by general practitioners (chapter fifteen). It may be that general practitioners, perceiving how stretched the service is, delay referral longer than they used to. On the other hand, nurses may have felt that they should be doing more for patients than they did in 1969. Some nurses were also critical of general practitioners for poor standards of pain control, which was generally somewhat worse at home than in hospital (chapter thirteen).

An alternative to exhorting general practitioners to make more home visits could be to give community nurses a more central role in the management of domiciliary care, so that relatives come to look to the nurse rather than the doctor as the key worker in this area. What this would require, however, is a delegation of the power traditionally held by doctors over decisions concerning pain control and other medication, over matters such as communicating and discussing diagnosis and prognosis, and over referral to specialist medical and nursing care, or hospital admissions. Community nurses visit the homes they go to more often than general practitioners, but at present they also visit fewer people at home in the last year of their lives, relying largely on general practitioners to identify those in need of care. Health visiting to monitor the condition of, perhaps, frail elderly people living alone, might become part of an extended role for community nurses.

It is, perhaps, significant that general practitioners, compared with consultants and district nurses, were the least welcoming to specialist domiciliary teams for terminal care (chapter sixteen). A few general practitioners clearly felt that these teams impinged on a job that should be their preserve. If such teams were to be extended to cover a broader clientele than just the terminally ill perhaps (as with the case of the MacMillan teams who sometimes have medical experts in palliative care attached) with some specialist medical input from geriatricians, they could fulfil a valuable role in countering the declining capacity of general practitioners to keep up with the need for home visiting amongst the elderly and those living alone.

Institutional care

Changes in the hospital service since 1969, involving shorter lengths of stay, more frequent admissions and discharges, and a greater proportion of deaths occurring in hospitals have clearly been reflected in the experiences of people in our study. With the greater frequency of admissions discharge arrangements assume a greater importance now than in 1969. Hospital staff have increasingly needed to learn how to refer patients to the community. In the light of this, it is encouraging to see that in spite of consultants sometimes demonstrating a lack of knowledge about available community services (chapter thirteen), district nurses felt that communication with hospital was better than they had in 1969 (chapter fifteen, Table 15.3). However, general practitioners were largely critical of the information given to them at discharge (chapter sixteen) so there is no room for complacency.

Hospital care is increasingly a place for acute care and short stays, and the balance of provision of long stay nursing facilities for the elderly has been shifting from the NHS to residential and nursing homes, particularly in the private sector (Table 1.7). The increased importance of these homes as a place of death justifies a degree of concern over their standards. More people (14 per cent) died in them than in hospices (4 per cent) in 1987

(Table 2.1), and the time spent living in such homes, with 54 per cent of residents having spent a year or more in such homes before their death (Table 11.1), is considerably greater than the time spent in any other form of institutional care. There was some evidence that the medical attention received by people in residential homes might have been improved, with a similar level of criticism of the lack of visiting by general practitioners as for people living in their own homes (chapter eleven). The desire for more generous facilities in some homes was evident (a telephone, single rooms, better food), but perhaps the most disturbing aspect was the situation of those who had few or no visitors in the last year of life. The loneliness of the dying (Elias 1985) is compounded by the loneliness of life before death for some of the very old.

Hospices

The growth of hospices in the years since the first study was, in part, an attempt to counter the loneliness of the person dying with cancer. A prevailing image in hospice literature is of such a person in a hospital, alone in a side ward, with poor emotional support and inadequate medical attention. The hospice movement has, undeniably, contributed to a reversal of the picture for people terminally ill with cancer. The results in chapter eight showed the considerable success of hospice care in relieving pain and in providing reassurance, support and medical and nursing care judged excellent by respondents. The role of specialist domiciliary nursing teams in this is clearly important and we have suggested that they might form a model for the wider domiciliary nursing service.

Causal relationships are difficult to establish in a descriptive survey, but the shift that has occurred in doctors' attitudes and practices in informing patients and relatives of diagnosis and prognosis in cancer (chapter three) has been largely in accord with hospice principles. However, as shown in chapter two, not all relatives were appreciative of the change. One limitation of the studies was that the views of the dying people themselves were not gathered and we cannot tell how they compared with the views of relatives. Relatives were more frequently given information about the prognosis than the dying people themselves (Table 3.6) and some people were left to guess things for themselves. Nurses, who have a greater involvement with the daily care of patients and their families than most doctors, are still rarely involved in communicating important medical information. There is still be work to do before this aspect of the loneliness of the dying can be said to be resolved.

Loneliness, and being alone at the end of life, is not just about fear of death, or embarrassment at facing bad news, important though these issues might be in terminal illness, or in bereavement and mourning (Gorer 1965). This study has shown to a considerable degree that the problems that face many in their last year of life are those of great age and its concomitant troubles, not just dying itself. The hospice movement has done a great deal to address the fears of the dying, but the travails of old age have increased since 1969. More people die when very old (chapter seven), living alone, or in institutional care (which may involve a deeper loneliness), increasingly needing care from others. The medical and social services available to the elderly could undergo a similar transformation to that provided by the hospice movement for people with terminal cancer, but clearly they have some way to go.

Caring for those with a terminal illness is often stressful and demanding; looking after those with chronic illness and the degenerative conditions of old age requires a longer term commitment. Both the 1969 and 1987 studies found that only one in ten deaths were sudden (chapter two), and as about a quarter of adult deaths are from cancer this leaves two thirds from conditions which are less likely to be clearly identified as terminal and more likely to be deaths of older people, associated with more long term restrictions and with less help available from relatives (chapter nine). The development of adequate services to meet the needs of this group presents an even greater challenge than that initially taken on by the hospice movement.

Bibliography

Abel, E.K. (1986), "The hospice movement: institutionalising innovation", *International Journal of Health Services,* 16, pp. 71-85.
Ahmedzai, S., Morton, A., Reid, J.T. and Stevenson, R.D. (1988), "Quality of death from lung cancer: patients' reports and relatives' retrospective opinions", In Watson, M., Greer, S. and Thomas, C., (eds). *Psychosocial Oncology,* Pergamon Press, Oxford.
Albery, N., Elliot, G. and Elliot, J. (Eds), (1993), *The Natural Death Handbook,* Virgin, London.
Aldridge, D.A. (1987), "A team approach to terminal care: personal implications for general practitioners", *Journal of the Royal College of General Practitioners,* 37, p. 364.
Allan, G. (1988), "Kinship, responsibility and care for elderly people", *Ageing and Society,* 8, pp. 249-68.
Allen, I., Hogg, D. and Peace, S. (1992), *Elderly people: choice, participation and satisfaction,* London, Policy Studies Institute.
Arber, S., Gilbert, N. (1988), "Men: the forgotten carers", *Sociology,* 23 (1), pp. 111-18.
Arber, S., Gilbert, G.N. and Evandrou, M. (1988), "Gender, household composition and receipt of domiciliary services by elderly disabled people", *Journal of Social Policy,* 17, pp. 153-75.
Arber, S. and Ginn, J. (1991), *Gender and Later Life: a sociological analysis of resources and constraints,* Sage, London and New York.
Aries, P. (1981), *The Hour of our Death,* Allen Lane, London.
Armstrong, D. (1987), "Silence and truth in death and dying", *Social Science and Medicine,* 24 (8), pp. 651-7.
Bebbington, A. and Tong, M. (1986), "Trends and changes in old people's homes: provision over twenty years", In Judge, K. and Sinclair, I. (eds) *Residential care for elderly people,* HMSO, London.

Berisa, F., McGonigle., R.J.S., Bearman, M., Michael, J. and Adu, D. (1989), "Chronic ambulatory peritoneal dialysis in patients over seventy", *Age and Ageing* 18, pp. 134-5.

Blackburn, A.M. (1989), "Problems of terminal care in elderly patients", *Palliative Medicine* 3, pp. 203-6.

Blane, D., Davey-Smith, G. and Bartley, M. (1990), "Social class differences in years of potential life lost: size, trends and principal causes", *British Medical Journal*, 301, pp. 429-32.

Bowling, A. and Cartwright, A. (1982), *Life after a death: a study of the elderly widowed,* Tavistock Publications, London and New York.

Bowling, A. (1983), "The hospitalisation of death: should more people die at home?", *Journal of Medical Ethics*, 9, pp. 158-61.

Brechling, B.G., Kuhn, D. (1989), "A specialised hospice for dementia patients and their families", *American Journal of Hospice Care,* May/June, pp. 27-30.

Brocklehurst, J.C. and Tucker, J.S. (1980), *Progress in Geriatric Day Care,* King's Fund, London.

Buchan, I.C. and Richardson, I.M. (1973), *Time study of consultations in general practice,* Scottish Health Studies, 27, Scottish Home and Health Department.

Butler, J.R. and Morgan, M. (1977), "Marital status and hospital use", *British Journal of Preventive and Social Medicine,* 31, 192-8.

Cartwright, A. (1970), *Parents and Family Planning Services,* Routledge and Kegan Paul, London and Boston.

Cartwright, A. (1990), "Medicine taking by people aged 65 or more", *British Medical Bulletin,* 46, pp. 63-76.

Cartwright, A. and Anderson, R. (1981), *General Practice Revisited,* Tavistock, London.

Cartwright, A., Hockey, L. and Anderson, J.L. (1973), *Life before death,* Routledge and Kegan Paul, London and Boston.

Cartwright, A. and O'Brien, M. (1976), "Social class variations in health care and in the nature of general practitioner consultations", In Stacey, M. (ed.) *The Sociology of the NHS,* Sociological Review Monograph No. 22.

Cartwright, A. and Seale, C. (1990), *The Natural History of a Survey: an account of the methodological issues encountered in a study of life before death,* King Edward's Hospital Fund, London.

Cartwright, A. and Smith, C. (1988), *Elderly People, their Medicines and their Doctors,* Routledge, London and New York.

Cathcart, F. (1988), "Seeing the body after death", *British Medical Journal,* 297, pp. 997-8.

Central Statistical Office. (1989), *Social Trends 19,* HMSO, London.

Chaggaris, M. and Lester, D. (1989), "Fear of death and religious belief", *Psychological Reports*, 64, p. 274.

Clench, P. (1984), *Managing to Care in Community Services for the Terminally Ill,* The Patten Press, Richmond.

Cook, C. and Hubner, P.J.B. (1989), "Percutaneous transluminal coronary angioplasty in elderly patients: a comparison with younger patients", *Age and Ageing*, 18, pp. 219-22.

Dale, A., Evandrou, M., Arber, S. (1987), "The household structure of the elderly population in Britain", *Ageing and Society*, 7, pp. 37-56.

Davey-Smith, G. Bartley, M. and Blane, D. (1990), "The Black report on socioeconomic inequalities in health 10 years on", *British Medical Journal*, 301, pp. 373-7.

Davis, J.A. and Jowell, R. (1989), "Measuring national differences: an introduction to the International Social Survey Programme", In Jowell, R., Witherspoon, S. and Brook, L. (eds) *British Social Attitudes: special international report,* Gower, London.

de Vaus, D.A. (1990), *Surveys in Social Research,* Unwin Hyman, London.

Department of Health (1988), *Health and Personal Social Services Statistics for England 1988,* HMSO, London.

Department of Health (1989), *Health and Personal Social Services Statistics for England 1989,* HMSO, London.

Department of Health (1990), *Health and Personal Social Services Statistics for England 1990,* HMSO, London.

Department of Health and Social Security (1973), *Health and Personal Social Services Statistics for England and Wales 1972,* HMSO, London.

Department of Health and Social Security (1977), *Health and Personal Social Services Statistics for England 1977,* HMSO, London.

Department of Health and Social Security (1978), *Health and Personal Social Services Statistics for England 1978,* HMSO, London.

Department of Health and Social Security (1982), *Health and Personal Social Services Statistics for England 1982,* HMSO, London.

Department of Health and Social Security (1987), *Residential accommodation for the elderly and for younger physically handicapped people: all residents in local authority, voluntary and private homes, RA/87/2,* HMSO, London.

Department of Health and Social Security, Research Working Group (1980), *Inequalities in Health,* HMSO, London.

Dixon, J.M. (1992), "Treatment of elderly patients with breast cancer", *British Medical Journal*, 304, pp. 996-7.

Donaldson, C., Wright, K.G., Maynard, A.K., Hamill, J.D., Sutcliffe, E. (1987), "Day hospitals for the elderly: utilisation and performance", *Community Medicine*, 9, pp. 55-61.

Downey, A.M. (1982), "Relationship of religiosity to death anxiety of middle aged males", *Psychological Reports,* 54, pp. 811-22.

Elias, N. (1985), *The Loneliness of the Dying,* Blackwell, Oxford.

Feifel, H. (1959), *The Meaning of Death,* McGraw-Hill, New York.

Feifel, H. and Branscomb, A.B. (1973), "Who's afraid of death?", *Journal of Abnormal Psychology,* 81, pp. 282-8.

Fennel, G. (1979), *Day centres for the elderly: an overview of three studies,* School of Economic and Social Studies, University of East Anglia.

Fentiman, I.S., Tirelli, U., Monfardini, S., Schneider, M., Festen, J., Cognetti, F. and Aapro, M.S. (1990), "Cancer in the elderly: why so badly treated?", *Lancet,* 335, pp. 1020-2.

Field, D. (1984), "We didn't want him to die on his own" - Nurses' accounts of nursing dying patients", *Journal of Advanced Nursing,* 9, pp. 59-70.

Field, D. (1989), *Nursing the Dying,* Tavistock/Routledge, London.

Fox, A.J., Goldblatt, P.O. and Jones, D.R. (1985), "Social class mortality differentials: artefact, selection or life circumstances?", *Journal of Epidemiology and Community Health,* 39, pp. 1-8.

Fry, J. (1983), "Deaths and dying", *Update,* 27 (12), pp. 1706-7.

Gilhooley, M.L.M., Berkeley, J., McCann, K., Gibling, F. and Murray, K. (1988), "Truth telling with dying cancer patients", *Palliative Medicine,* 2, pp. 64-71.

Glaser, B.G. and Strauss, A.L. (1965), *Awareness of Dying,* Aldine, Chicago.

Goffman, E. (1961), *Asylums: essays on the social situation of mental patients and other inmates,* Doubleday, New York

Gorer, G. (1955), "The pornography of death", *Encounter,* 5, pp. 49-53.

Gorer, G. (1965), *Death, Grief and Mourning,* Cresset, London.

Gray, D.J.P. (1978), "Feeling at home", *Journal of the Royal College of General Practitioners,* 28, pp. 6-17.

Haig, R., Castleden, M., Woods, K., Fletcher, S., Bowns, I., Gibson, M. and Soper, J. (1991), "Management of myocardial infarction in the elderly: admission and outcome on a coronary care unit", *Health Trends,* 23, pp. 154-7.

Haines, A. and Booroff, A. (1986), "Terminal care at home: perspective from general practice", *British Medical Journal,* 292, pp. 1051-3.

Hammersley, M. and Atkinson, P. (1983) *Ethnography: principles in practice,* Tavistock, London.

Henderson, J., Goldacre, M.J., and Griffith, M. (1990), "Hospital care for the elderly in the final year of life: a population based study", *British Medical Journal,* 301, pp. 17-19.

Higginson, I., McCarthy, M. (1989), "Evaluation of palliative care: steps to quality assurance?", *Palliative Medicine,* 3, pp. 267-74.

Hinton, J.M. (1963), "The physical and mental distress of the dying", *Quarterly Journal of Medicine,* 32 (1), pp.   .

Hinton, J. (1967), *Dying,* Penguin Books, Harmondsworth.

Hinton, J.M. (1979), "Comparison of places and policies for terminal care", *Lancet,* 1, pp. 29-32.

Hughes, H.L.G. (1960), *Peace at Last,* Calouste Gulbenkian Foundation, London.

Isaacs, B., Livingstone, M. and Neville, Y. (1972), *Survival of the Unfittest: a study of geriatric patients in Glasgow London and Boston,* Routledge and Kegan Paul, London and Boston.

Jacoby, A. (1990), "Management strategies and patient needs: the provision of nursing care in the community", *Journal of Advanced Nursing,* vol.15, pp.1409-17.

James, N. and Field, D. (1992) "The routinization of hospice: charisma and bureaucratization", *Social Science and Medicine,* 34 (12), pp. 1363-75.

Jefferys, M. and Thane, P. (1989), "An ageing society and ageing people", In Jefferys, M. (ed.), *Growing Old in the Twentieth Century,* Routledge, London and New York.

Johnson, P. (1989), "The structured dependency of the elderly: a critical note", In Jefferys, M. (ed.), *Growing Old in the Twentieth Century,* Routledge, London and New York.

Joint National Cancer Survey Committee, (1952), *Report on a national survey concerning patients with cancer nursed at home,* Marie Curie Memorial, London.

Judge, K. and Sinclair, I. (1986), *Residential care for elderly people,* HMSO, London.

Kane, R.L., Wales, J., Bernstein, L., Leibowitz, A. and Kaplon, S. "A randomised controlled trial of hospice care", *Lancet,* 1, pp. 890-4.

Kubler-Ross, E. (1970), *On Death and Dying,* Macmillan, New York.

Laing, W. (1985), *Private health care 1985,* Office of Health Economics, London.

Lancet. (1980), "In cancer honesty is here to stay", *Lancet,* vol.ii, p. 245.

Lancet. (1986), "Hospice comes of age", *Lancet,* pp. 1013-14.
3 May 1986

Levin, E., Sinclair, I.A.C., and Gorbach, P. (1983), *Supporters of Confused Elderly Persons at Home,* National Institute for Social Work, London.

Levin, E., Sinclair, I.A.C. and Gorbach, P. (1989), *Families, Services and Confusion in Old Age,* Gower, London.

Lewis, J. and Meredith, B. (1988), "Daughters caring for mothers: the experience of caring and its implications for professional helpers", *Ageing and Society,* 8, pp. 1-21.

Lewis, J. and Meredith, B. (1989), "Contested territory in informal care", In Jefferys, M. (ed.), *Growing Old in the Twentieth Century,* Routledge, London and New York.

Lunt, B. (1985), *A comparison of hospice and hospital care for terminally ill cancer patients and their families,* Unpublished report to the Department of Health and Social Security, University of Southampton.

Lunt, B. and Hillier, R. (1981), "Terminal care: present services and future priorities", *British Medical Journal,* 283, pp. 595-8.

Lunt, B. and Yardley, J. (1986), *A survey of home care teams and hospital support teams for the terminally ill,* Unpublished report, Cancer Care Research Unit, Royal South Hampshire Hospital, 1986.

MacDonald, L. and MacNair, R. (1986), "Your views on terminal care", *Journal of District Nursing,* 4(9), p. 1986.

McCardie, W.R. (1981), "Religiosity and fear of death: strength of belief systems", *Psychological Reports,* 49, pp. 921-2.

McIntosh, J. (1977), *Communication and Awareness on a Cancer Ward,* Croom Helm, London.

Maguire, P. and Faulkner, A. (1988), "How to do it: Improve the counselling skills of doctors and nurses in cancer care",
British Medical Journal, 297, pp. 847-9.

Mahoney, J.J. (1986), "Lessons from hospice evaluation: counterpoints", *The Hospice Journal,* 2, pp. 9-15.

Martin, B. (1990), "The cultural construction of ageing: or How long can the summer wine actually last?", In Bury, M. and MacNicol, J. (eds), *Aspects of Ageing,* Social Policy Papers No. 3, Department of Social Policy, Royal Holloway and Bedford New College, London.

Mor, V. (1987), *Hospice Care Systems: structure, process, costs, and outcomes,* Springer, New York.

Morris, J.N. (1990), "Inequalities in health: ten years and a little further on", *Lancet,* 336, pp. 491-3.

Moser, C.A. and Kalton, G. (1971), *Survey methods in social investigation,* Heinemann Books, London.

Muchnik, B. and Rosenheim, E. (1982), "Fear of death, defense style and religiosity among Israeli jews", *The Israel Journal of Psychiatry and Related Sciences,* 19, pp. 157-64.

National Hospice Study. (1986), *Journal of Chronic Disease,* 39 (1).

Neill, J., Sinclair, I., Gorbach, P. and Williams, J. (1988), *A Need for Care? Elderly applicants for local authority homes,* Gower, London.

Novack, D.H., Plumer, R., Smith, R.L., Ochitill, H., Morrow, G.R. and Bennett, J.M. (1979), "Changes in physicians' attitudes toward telling the cancer patient", *Journal of the American Medical Association,* 241, pp.

897-900.
Office of Health Economics (1992), *Compendium of Health Statistics,* 8th edition, Office of Health Economics, London.
Office of Population Censuses and Surveys (1975) *General Household Survey 1972,* HMSO, London.
Office of Population Censuses and Surveys (1977), *Population Trends 10,* HMSO, London.
Office of Population Censuses and Surveys (1980) *Classification of occupations,* HMSO, London.
Office of Population Censuses and Surveys (1982) *General Household Survey 1980,* HMSO, London.
Office of Population Censuses and Surveys (1987), *Mortality Statistics: Cause 1987,* HMSO, London.
Office of Population Censuses and Surveys (1989), *Mortality Statistics 1986,* HMSO, London.
Office of Population Censuses and Surveys (1989) *General Household Survey 1987,* HMSO, London.
Office of Population Censuses and Surveys (1991) *General Household Survey 1989,* HMSO, London.
Office of Population Censuses and Surveys (1992a), *Mortality Statistics, General. Review of the Registrar General on deaths in England & Wales 1990,* HMSO, London.
Office of Population Censuses and Surveys (1992b), *Population Trends 69,* HMSO, London.
Office of Population Censuses and Surveys (1993), *Population Trends 71,* HMSO, London.
Oken, D. (1961), "What to tell cancer patients: a study of medical attitudes", *Journal of the American Medical Association,* 175, pp. 1120-8.
Ormerod, O.J.M. and Westaby, S. (1988), "Interventional cardiology and cardiac surgery in the elderly", In Grimley Evans, J. and Caird, F.I. (eds) *Advanced Geriatric Medicine,* 7, pp. 38-49.
Parkes, C.M. (1972), *Bereavement: studies of grief in adult life,* Penguin Books, Harmondsworth.
Parkes, C.M. (1979a), "Terminal care: evaluation of an in-patient service at St Christopher's Hospice, Part 1: Views of surviving spouse on effect of the service on the patient", *Postgraduate Medical Journal,* 55, pp. 517-22.
Parkes, C.M. (1979b), "Self-assessments of the effects of the service on surviving spouses", *Postgraduate Medical Journal,* 55, pp. 523-7.
Parkes, C.M. (1980), "Terminal care: evaluation of an advisory domiciliary service at St Christopher's Hospice", *Postgraduate Medical Journal,* 56, pp. 685-9.

Parkes, C.M. (1981), "Evaluation of a bereavement service", *Journal of Preventive Psychiatry,* 1, pp. 179-88.

Parkes, C.M. and Parkes, J. (1984), ""Hospice" versus "Hospital" care - re-evaluation after ten years as seen by surviving spouses", *Postgraduate Medical Journal,* 60, pp. 120-4.

Parkes, C.M. (1985), "Terminal care: home, hospital or hospice?", *Lancet,* i, pp. 155-7.

Pell, A.C.H., Stuart, P.C., Stewart, M.J. and Fraser, D.M. (1990), "Home or hospital care for acute myocardial infarction? A survey of general practitioners' attitudes in the thrombolytic era", *The British Journal of General Practice,* 40, pp. 323-5.

Prior, L. (1989), *The Social Organization of Death: medical discourses and social practices in Belfast,* MacMillan, Basingstoke and London.

Qureshi, H. Walker, A. (1989), The Caring Relationship: elderly people and their families", MacMillan, Basingstoke and London.

Rees, W.D. (1972), "The distress of dying", *British Medical Journal,* 3, pp. 105-7.

Rees, W.D. (1982), "Role of the hospice in the care of the dying", *British Medical Journal,* 285, pp. 1766-8.

Registrar General (1969), *The Registrar General's Statistical Review of England and Wales for the Year 1969,* Part1: Medical, HMSO, London.

Rose, N (1989) *Governing the Soul: The shaping of the private self,* Routledge, London and New York.

Royal College of General Practitioners, Office of Population Censuses and Surveys and Department of Health and Social Security (1990), *Morbidity statistics from general practice, third national study, socio-economic analyses,* 1981-82 Series MB5 No. 2. HMSO, London.

St Christopher's Hospice Information Service, (1987) *1987 Directory of Hospice Services,* Hospice Information Service, London.

St Christopher's Hospice Information Service, (1993) *1993 Directory of Hospice Services,* Hospice Information Service, London.

Saunders, C.M. (1978), (ed.), *The Management of Terminal Disease,* Edward Arnold, London.

Saunders, C.M. and Baines, M. (1983), *Living with Dying: the management of terminal disease,* Oxford University Press, Oxford, New York, Toronto.

Seale, C.F. (1989), "What happens in hospices: a review of research evidence", *Social Science and Medicine,* 28 (6), pp. 551-9.

Secretaries of State for Health, Social Security, Wales and Scotland (1989), *Caring for People: community care in the next decade and beyond,* HMSO, London.

Simms, M. (1984), "Taking the strain?", *Senior Nurse,* 1 (34), pp. 21-2.

Standing Medical Advisory Committee, (1980), *Terminal Care: Report of a Working Group,* HMSO, London.

Sudnow, D. (1967), *Passing On: the social organization of dying,* Prentice-Hall, New Jersey.

Svenson, W. (1961), "Attitudes towards death in an aged population", *Journal of Gerontology,* 16, pp. 49-52.

Taylor, H. (1983), *The Hospice Movement in Britain: its role and future,* Centre for Policy on Ageing, London.

Tester, S. (1989), *Caring by day,* Centre for Policy on Ageing, London.

Timaeus, I. (1986), "Families and households of the elderly population: prospects for those approaching old age", *Ageing and Society,* 6, pp. 271-93.

Tuffnel, G. and Warburton, R.W. (1981), "Elderly users of day care: a census of old people attending grade "A" day centres in Cambridgeshire", *Clearing house for local authority social services research,* 6, pp. 27-36.

Twycross, R. (1978), "Relief of pain", In Saunders, C.M. (ed.), *The Management of Terminal Disease,* Edward Arnold, London.

Victor, C. (1991), *Health and Health Care in Later Life,* Open University Press, Milton Keynes and Philadelphia.

Wadsworth, M.E.J., Sinclair, S. and Wirz, H.M. (1972), "A geriatric day hospital and its system of care", *Social Science and Medicine,* 6, pp. 507-25.

Ward, A.W.M. (1974), "Telling the patient", *Journal of the Royal College of General Practitioners,* 24, pp. 465-8.

Ward, A.W.M. (1985), *Home Care Services for the Terminally Ill: a report for the Nuffield Foundation,* University of Sheffield, Department of Community Medicine.

Weaver, T., Willcocks, D. and Kellaher, L. (1985), *The Business of Care: a study of private residential homes for old people,* Report No. 1, The Polytechnic of North London, Centre for Environmental and Social Studies in Ageing.

West, S.R., Harris, B.J., Warren, A., Wood, H., Montgomery, B. and Belsham, V. (1986), "A retrospective study of patients with cancer in their terminal year", *New Zealand Medical Journal,* 99, pp. 197-200.

Wilkes, E. (1965), "Terminal cancer at home" *Lancet,* i, pp. 799-801.

Wilkes, E. (1984), *A Source Book of Terminal Care,* Sheffield University Press, Sheffield.

Wilkin, D. and Hughes, B. (1987), "Residential care of elderly people: the consumers' views", *Ageing and Society,* 7, pp. 175-201.

Williams, A. (1990), "Incurable illness", *British Medical Journal,* 301, p. 67.

Williams, E.I. and Fitton, F. (1990), "General practitioner response to elderly patients discharged from hospital", *British Medical Journal,* 300, pp. 159-61.

Wilson. J,A, Lawson, P.M. and Smith, R.G. (1987), "The treatment of terminally ill geriatric patients", *Palliative Medicine,* 1, pp. 149-53

Worden, J.W. (1991), *Grief Counselling and Grief Therapy: a handbook for the mental health practitioner,* Tavistock/Routledge, London and New York.

Copyright acknowledgements

We gratefully acknowledge permission to reprint material from the following sources:

Chapter 2: reprinted from Cartwright, A. (1991), "Changes in life and care in the year before death 1969-1987", *Journal of Public Health Medicine,* 13, 2, pp. 81-87, with kind permission from Oxford University Press.

Chapter 3: reprinted from Seale, C.F. (1991), "Communication and awareness about death: a study of a random sample of dying people", *Social Science and Medicine,* 32, 8, pp. 943-952, with kind permission from Pergamon Press Ltd, Headington Hill Hall, Oxford, OX3 OBW, UK.

Chapter 4: reprinted from Cartwright, A. (1991), "Is religion a help around the time of death?", *Public Health,* 105, pp. 79-87, with kind permission from the Society of Public Health.

Chapter 5: reprinted from Seale, C.F. (1990), "Caring for people who die: the experience of family and friends", *Ageing and Society,* 10, 4, pp. 413-428, with kind permission from Cambridge University Press.

Chapter 6: reprinted from Cartwright, A. (1992), "Social class differences in health and care in the year before death", *Journal of Epidemiology and Community health,* 46, 1, pp. 54-57, with kind permission from the British Medical Association.

Chapter 7: reprinted from Cartwright, A. (1993) "Dying when you're old", *Age and Ageing,* 22, pp. 425-30 with kind permission from Oxford University Press.

Chapter 8: reprinted from Seale, C.F. (1991), "A comparison of hospice and conventional care", *Social Science and Medicine,* 32, 2, pp. 147-152, with kind permission from Pergamon Press Ltd, Headington Hill Hall, Oxford, OX3 OBW, UK.

Chapter 9: reprinted from Seale, C.F. (1991), "Death from cancer and death from other causes: the relevance of the hospice approach", *Palliative Medicine,* 5, pp. 12-19, with kind permission from Edward Arnold, Hodder and Stoughton Educational.

Chapter 10: reprinted from Cartwright, A. (1991) "The role of hospitals in caring for people in the last year of their lives", *Age and Ageing,* 20, pp. 271-4, with kind permission from Oxford University Press.

Chapter 11: reprinted from Cartwright, A. (1991), "The role of residential and nursing homes in the last year of people's lives", *British Journal of Social Work,* 21, pp. 627-645, with kind permission from Oxford University Press.

Chapter 12: reprinted from Farrow, G. (1992), "The role of day centres in caring for people in the final year of their lives", *Ageing and Society,* 12, pp. 313-327, with kind permission from Cambridge University Press.

Chapter 13: reprinted from Cartwright, A. (1991), "Balance of care for the dying between hospitals and the community: perceptions of general practitioners, hospital consultants, community nurses and relatives", *British Journal of General Practice,* 41, pp. 271-274, with kind permission from the Royal College of General Practitioners.

Chapter 14: reprinted from Cartwright, A. (1990), *The role of the general practitioner in caring for people in the last year of their lives,* King Edward's Hospital Fund for London, with kind permission from the Institute for Social Studies in Medical Care.

Chapter 15: reprinted from Seale, C.F. (1992), "Community nurses and the care of the dying", *Social Science and Medicine,* 34, 4, pp. 375-382, with kind permission from Pergamon Press Ltd, Headington Hill Hall, Oxford, OX3 OBW, UK.

Chapter 16: reprinted from Cartwright, A. (1991), "The relationship between general practitioners, hospital consultants and community nurses when caring for people in the last year of their lives", *Family Practice,* 8, pp. 350-355, with kind permission from Oxford University Press.

Index

Abel, K.K. 8
acceptance of death 46-7, 56-7, 61, 121
age, effects of 89-93, 125, 132, 134-5, 145, 148, 155, 177
Ahmedzai, S. 109
Albery, N. 8
amenities in residential homes 80, 139-40
Arber, S. 3, 62, 67, 219
Aries, P. 9
Armstrong, D. 31
awareness
 attitudes of professionals 9, 348, 204, 206, 210-11, 217
 changes 1969-1987 24-8, 39, 42-4, 50, 110
 of diagnosis 25, 39-41, 102-3, 204
 of dying 9, 39-41, 51, 84, 110, 119-21
 preferences of respondents 26, 45-8, 178
 source of information 42-4, 48-9

bereavement 9, 32, 59, 61, 72-6, 108-11, 122-123, 219, 224
 counselling 185-8, 193, 207

Blackburn, A.M. 112, 120-1, 123
Bowling, A. 35, 61, 71, 108-9, 189
cancer
 and age 62, 87, 127
 and awareness 27-8, 39, 103
 and care at home 67
 and dying alone 71-2
 and general practitioner consultations 175-6
 and hospice care 8-9, 101-2, 105, 128, 223
 and nursing management 197
 and pain control 166, 205
 and symptoms 101-2, 126
carers
 experience of caring 75-6, 118, 154
 relief from caring 147, 154, 158-9
 and social isolation 70
 stress of caring 68-70, 122, 220, 224
 support for 197
 who they are 67-8
Cartwright, A. 10, 13-14, 22, 35, 61, 81-2, 90, 109, 110, 130, 134, 148, 152, 189, 194, 197

changes 1969-1987 2-13, 18-28, 39, 48, 63, 66-7, 75, 124, 127, 163-4, 195 202 207 219-24
chiropody 6, 118, 147, 152, 158, 164, 197, 221
closed awareness 8, 9, 35, 40-1, 51
community nurses 195-209
   attitudes to communication 35, 201, 213, 217, 218
   changes in service provision 6, 22, 163-4, 166-70, 197, 217, 221-2
   and pain control 172-3, 217
   specialists in terminal care 214-7
conspiracy of silence
   see closed awareness
consultants *see* hospital doctors

day centres 16, 92, 98, 147-59, 163
demographic change 2-4, 6, 32, 33, 68, 75, 89, 113, 219-20
Department of Health 4-7, 127, 185
Department of Health and Social Security 4-7, 130-1, 177
disability *see* restrictions
district nursing
   see community nurses

Elias, N. 9-10, 32, 223
emotional reactions to death and dying
   of general practitioners 28, 35, 186-8, 193
   of hospital doctors 35, 51
   of nurses 35, 206

Feifel, H. 9, 52
Field, D. 37
financial resources 77, 83-5, 131

General Household Survey 5, 62
gender differences
   and age 2-3, 89, 113, 122, 132-3, 148-9
   and bereavement 73-4
   and caring 62, 67, 75-6, 219
   and general practitioner consultations 177-8
   and living alone 62-5, 75, 76, 150, 219
   and place of death 127
   and religious faith 54, 55, 57, 59, 60
general practitioners 175-94, 220
   attitudes towards training 28, 185, 193, 216
   changes 1969-1987 4-5, 21-2, 26, 163-4
   and home nurses 37-8, 195, 203, 206, 212-3, 215, 218
   and home visiting 22, 27, 74, 81, 92, 119, 136-7, 163-4, 173, 176-7, 189, 193-4, 220
   and hospices 170
   and hospitals 128-9, 168, 170-1, 210-2, 217
   and night calls 119, 136, 145, 175-7
   and pain control 171-3, 205
   and residential homes 136-7, 145
Glaser, B.G. 9, 10, 35, 40
Goffman, E. 10
Gorer, G. 9, 224
grief *see* bereavement

Higginson, I. 109
Hinton, J.M. 35, 32, 100
home help 6, 22-4, 68, 91, 154-5, 157-9, 163-4, 167-8, 170, 221
hospices 97-123, 223-4
   growth of 1, 97
   and the non cancer patient 87,

101-2, 112, 122-3
  numbers served by 97-8, 101, 124-5
  philosophy of 8-10, 119-20
hospital doctors
  and domiciliary consultations 211-2
  views of community care 166-9, 173
  views on pain control 171-2
hospitals
  admission 170
  admittance from residential homes 137-9, 145
  changes 1969-1987 7, 20-1, 124, 222
  length of stay 7, 20, 85, 124-5, 168
  relatives' views 72, 127-8, 171-3
household composition 20, 62-8, 148-9
housing 83, 91

incontinence 24, 27, 66, 82, 89, 134-5, 142, 145, 212 219
information
  about death and illness 24-6, 34-51, 84, 223
  given to general practitioners 210, 217, 222
  given to nurses 203-5, 213

Jacoby, A. 22
Jefferys, M. 145

Kane, R.L. 109
Kubler-Ross, E. 9, 31

Life before death, 1969 survey 10-15, 67, 97, 163
living alone 3, 14, 24, 27, 62-5, 92

loneliness 223-4
Lunt, B. 1, 100, 195

McIntosh, J. 35
MacMillan nurses 195, 196, 210, 222
  see also community nurses
Maguire, P. 34, 38
Mahoney, J.J. 109
Marie Curie sitters
  see night sitting service
meals on wheels 6, 70, 164
mental confusion
  and age 27, 66, 82, 89, 118, 134
  and awareness 41, 51
  and duration 24, 27, 66, 116, 134
  and information at referral 205
  and institutional care 65, 134, 135, 145
  long term 41, 116, 118, 122, 123, 152, 219
  respondents' accounts 110
Mor, V. 205
mourning *see* bereavement

National Hospice Study 100, 108
night sitting services 168-9, 173, 212, 213, 221
Novack, D.H. 34
nursing homes
  see residential homes

old peoples' homes
  see residential homes
open communication 27-8, 31, 34, 38, 40, 42, 46, 48, 50-1, 110
over treatment 128, 171, 218

pain
  control of 8, 37, 110, 128, 164,

166, 171-4, 205, 221-2, 223
experience of 24, 28, 66, 71, 102, 106, 113, 116, 118, 122, 134, 181, 183-4
training in management of 207, 216, 217
palliative medicine 8, 32, 105-6, 112, 212, 222
Parkes, C.M. 8, 32, 100, 109, 166
physiotherapy 147, 153
place of death 7, 15, 20-1, 32, 49, 63, 71-2, 80, 97, 98, 101-2, 106-8, 112, 124, 126-7, 130, 166, 172-3, 183, 175-6, 222
poverty 3, 77, 85
Prior, L. 9

psychotherapy 31

quality of life 8, 13, 71, 84-5, 143-4, 219

Rees, W.D. 35, 101
religion 31-2, 37, 52-61, 74, 101-2, 109, 206
residential homes 130-46, 222-3
and age 65, 89, 125, 132-3, 155
changes in provision 7
private 7, 80, 85, 130-1, 140, 222-3
and social class 80
response rates 13-15, 173, 197
restrictions 63-7, 77, 82, 84-5, 89, 91-2, 102, 103, 113, 117-19, 122, 150-2, 154-8, 224
room
(patient's), in hospital 81, 106
in hospice 106
(of one's own), in residential home 80, 139, 223

St Christopher's Hospice 1, 8, 100-1, 109
Directory of Hospice Services 100
sampling 10, 13, 101-2
Saunders, C.M. 8, 75-6, 81, 105, 106, 112, 197
Seale, C.F. 10, 13-14, 62, 90, 100, 109-10, 197
seeing the body 108
sex differences
see gender differences
Simms, M. 164, 197, 205, 208, 218
social class 77-85
and general practitioner's care 182
and general practitioner consultations 177
and hospice patients 102
and religious belief 55
study areas 13
Sudnow, D. 10
sudden death 18, 72
symptoms
and age 89-90, 93, 148
related to bereavement 109
and cancer 113, 116, 118, 122, 126
changes 1969-1987 24, 66
of those attending day centres 151-2, 156
of hospice patients 102
relief from 106, 110, 203, 214-6
of those in residential homes 134-5, 145
and social class 82
training in relief of 187

Taylor, H. 166
terminal care and non cancer patients 112
timeliness of death 71-2, 84, 121,

122-3
training 28, 34, 173, 185, 187-9, 191, 193, 199, 216
  for nurses 206-7, 217
Twycross, R. 8, 164

unexpected death *see* sudden death
unmet need 11, 91, 93, 218, 221

views about care received
  from general practitioners 178-84
  from hospital doctors 107
  from nurses 103-4, 107
visits
  to day centres 153-4, 158
  from relatives 70, 112, 142-3, 146, 223
  from nurses 103, 119, 139, 154, 169, 196-7, 199-200, 207
  professionals to the bereaved 74, 108-9
  respondents to hospices and hospitals 106
  see also general practioners and home visits; and night calls
  see also hospital doctors and domiciliary consultations

Ward, A.W.M. 35, 63, 67, 104, 110, 195, 197
Wilkes, E. 35, 67

year before death in 1987, The 11-15